HANDBOOK OF OPHTHALMOLOGIC EMERGENCIES

HANDBOOK OF OPHTHALMOLOGIC EMERGENCIES

THIRD EDITION

Edited by

Alfonse A. Cinotti, M.D., F.A.C.S.
Professor and Chairman
Department of Ophthalmology
University of Medicine and Dentistry
of New Jersey–New Jersey Medical School
Medical Director
Eye Institute of New Jersey
Newark, New Jersey

MEDICAL EXAMINATION PUBLISHING COMPANY

Main entry under title:

Handbook of ophthalmologic emergencies.

Rev. ed. of: Handbook of ophthalmologic emergencies/ by George M. Gombos. 2nd ed. c1977.
Includes bibliographies and index.
1. Ophthalmologic emergencies--Handbooks, manuals, etc. I. Cinotti, Alfonse A. II. Gombos, George M., (date) . Handbook of ophthalmologic emergencies.
[DNLM: 1. Emergencies--handbooks. 2. Ophthalmology--handbooks. WW 39 H236]
RE48.H28 1985 617.7'026 85-2891
ISBN 0-87488-532-9

ELSEVIER SCIENCE PUBLISHING COMPANY, INC.
52 Vanderbilt Avenue
New York, N.Y. 10017

Printed in the United States of America

Contents

Appendices

Contributors

JAMES V. BASTEK, M. D., Clinical Assistant Professor of Ophthalmology, UMDNJ-New Jersey Medical School, Newark, NJ

FRANCIS E. CANGEMI, M. D., Clinical Associate Professor of Ophthalmology, UMDNJ-New Jersey Medical School, Newark, NJ

DONALD J. CINOTTI, M. D., Clinical Instructor of Ophthalmology, UMDNJ-New Jersey Medical School, Newark, NJ

WILLIAM F. GRANT, M. D., Associate Professor of Clinical Ophthalmology and Clinical Preventive Medicine, UMDNJ-New Jersey Medical School, Newark, NJ

ROBERT C. HARBOUR, M. D., Head Fellow in Neuroophthalmology, Temple University School of Medicine, Philadelphia, PA

BARRY A. MALTZMAN, M. D., Clinical Associate Professor of Ophthalmology, UMDNJ-New Jersey Medical School, Newark, NJ

JOSEPH A. MAURIELLO, Jr., M. D., Assistant Professor of Ophthalmology, UMDNJ-New Jersey Medical School, Newark, NJ

MARK L. MOSTER, M. D., Assistant Professor of Neurology, Temple University School of Medicine, Philadelphia, PA

RUDOLPH S. WAGNER, M. D., Assistant Professor of Ophthalmology, UMDNJ-New Jersey Medical School, Newark, NJ

JAMES H. WHITE, M. D., F. R. C. S., Clinical Professor of Ophthalmology, UMDNJ-New Jersey Medical School, Newark, NJ

Preface

This is the third revision of Handbook of Ophthalmologic Emergencies. The collection was first compiled by George Gombos, M. D. with the help of his collaborators Peter Ballen, M. D., George Herman, M. D., Richard C. Troutman, M. D., and Arthur H. Wolintz, M. D.

The original purpose of this handbook was to provide guidance in ophthalmology for emergency room physicians and residents. The material has so well fulfilled that initial purpose, that in bringing out the third edition we have made only small changes in the basic material. Wherever necessary, we have included up-to-date techniques in evaluating and treating ocular emergencies. To that end we have added a chapter on Pediatric Eye Emergencies and appendices on Evaluation of Ocular Complaints or Symptoms and on Commonly Used Drugs in Ophthalmology.

Acknowledgments

The editor and authors would like to thank the following people for their help in the preparation of this work: for editorial assistance – Barbara A. Fitzgerald, C. O. T., Program Director of Ophthalmic Allied Health Programs at UMDNJ - New Jersey Medical School, Newark, New Jersey; for technical assistance – Delma M. Morales, secretary in the Department of Ophthalmology at UMDNJ - New Jersey Medical School, Newark, New Jersey; and for photography – Richard N. Press, C. R. A., medical photographer at the Eye Institute of New Jersey, Newark, New Jersey.

notice

Chapter 1

EYE EXAMINATION

The routine emergency room examination of the patient with an eye problem should include the following: history, physical examination, and special examinations.

HISTORY

Careful history, including general information, is very important in an attempt to reach the correct diagnosis and provide appropriate treatment. Routine questions, such as the patient's age and general health, should not be neglected under any circumstances. Very often, these questions may lead to useful information. Other helpful information should be obtained, such as:

1. Allergies to drugs
2. Immunization to tetanus
3. Past eye diseases or injuries
4. A family history of eye diseases and blindness
5. In the case of an injury, a history of the accident.

The most important symptoms to be elicited are:

1. Visual impairment
2. Pain or discomfort
3. Red eye
4. Double vision
5. Discharge or secretions

There are many more specific symptoms which may help make a diagnosis. These include visual and nonvisual ocular symptoms. A list of these various symptoms may be found in Appendix I.

PHYSICAL EXAMINATION

Physical examination of the eye should include the following: (1) visual acuity, (2) inspection of the external ocular structures including eyelids and lacrimal apparatus, (3) position of the eye and eye movements, (4) pupils, (5) intraocular pressure, (6) visual fields, and (7) ophthalmoscopy.

VISUAL ACUITY

The most important single test of ocular function is the evaluation of visual acuity. This examination should be an integral part of the eye examination of all patients who are able to give reliable subjective responses.

Various types of letter charts are available to examine visual acuity. The Snellen chart is one of the more commonly used (Fig. 1-1). The chart is usually placed 20 feet from the patient. Under difficult technical circumstances, the chart could be placed 15 feet from the patient. The chart should be illuminated. Approximately 100-foot candles provide adequate illumination.

Acuity is recorded as a fraction. The numerator represents the distance to the chart and the denominator represents the distance at which a normal eye can read the line. Therefore, 20/200 indicates that the patient is 20 feet away and can read the line that a normal eye can read at 200 feet. Preschool children or illiterates should be tested with an illiterate E chart (Fig. 1-2). For this test, the patient is taught to point his finger in the direction of the E bars.

Visual acuity is examined one eye at a time. The other eye should be occluded. Pressure on the occluded eye should be avoided. The patient is asked to read with one eye as far down the chart as possible. This is recorded and the same procedure is repeated for the other eye.

If the patient wears glasses for distance vision, the test is repeated with glasses. The result should be recorded as "corrected visual acuity." The result without glasses is recorded as "uncorrected visual acuity." When visual acuity is diminished, even with glasses, the test may be done with a pinhole. If the patient's vision is improved through the pinhole to nearly normal, it may be an indication that the impairment is due to a refractive error.

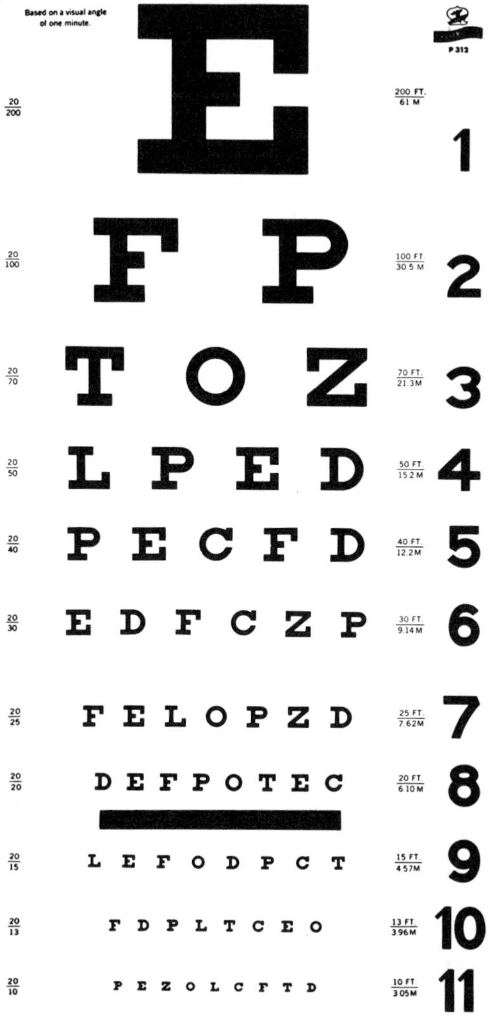

Fig. 1-1. Visual acuity chart, based on a visual angle of 1 minute.

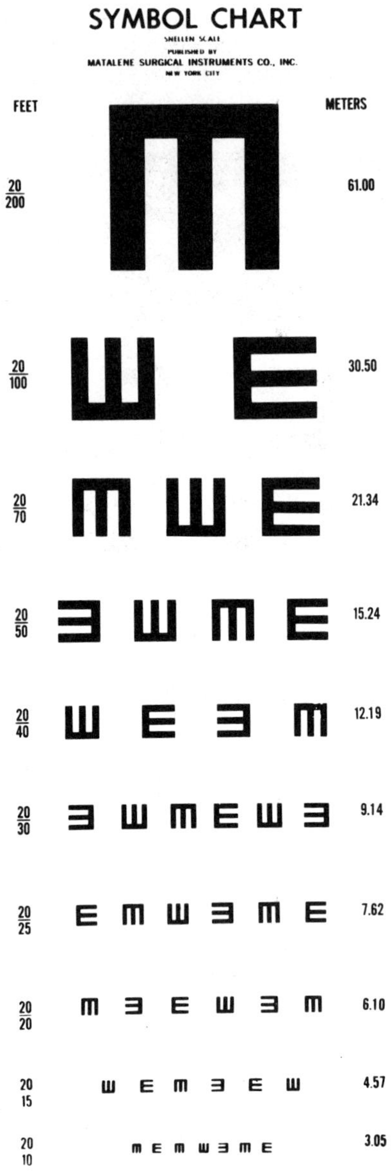

Fig. 1-2. Visual acuity chart for preschool children or illiterates.

The patient may be moved closer to the chart when unable to read the largest letter and the acuity recorded as the distance from the chart over the letter read, e. g. , 10/200. The ability to count fingers at a close distance may also be used, e. g. , cf/ 2 feet. Poorer visual acuity is recorded as light perception and, when the patient is able to indicate the position of the light in four quadrants, as light projection. If the patient is unable to see light, it is recorded as no light perception or NLP.

Measurement of near vision may be substituted when distance charts are not available. The test should be performed with glasses, especially for those patients in the presbyopic age (Fig. 1-3). In an emergency any reading material may be used to determine whether vision is impaired.

INSPECTION OF THE EXTERNAL OCULAR STRUCTURES

Inspection of the external ocular structures should include the lids (upper and lower), the lacrimal apparatus (gland, canaliculi, lacrimal sac), conjunctivas, corneas and scleras. The examination is greatly facilitated by use of a well-focused source of light and a magnifying loop or slit lamp.

The Lids

The important objectives of lid examination are: (1) detection of local disease or injury, (2) detection of local signs of systemic diseases, and (3) inspection of the physiologic functions of the eyelids.

Lid infection, retention cyst of the meibomian gland, traumatic wound of the eyelid, or infection of the lacrimal sac are only a few examples of local diseases to be detected by physical examination. Periorbital edema may indicate allergy or systemic diseases of the heart, kidney, or thyroid. Ptosis, drooping of the upper lid, may be congenital or acquired. The latter may suggest local eye diseases, third nerve palsies or myasthenia gravis; abnormal position of the lid border can be a frequent cause of eye irritation. Eversion of the lid (ectropion) can cause annoying tearing. Inversion of the lid (entropion) produces irritation by the lashes rubbing against the cornea and conjunctiva.

The meibomian glands may be seen on the margins of both lids. Blockage of one or more of these glands may produce swelling of the lid, pain, and tenderness (chalazion). Abnormal position

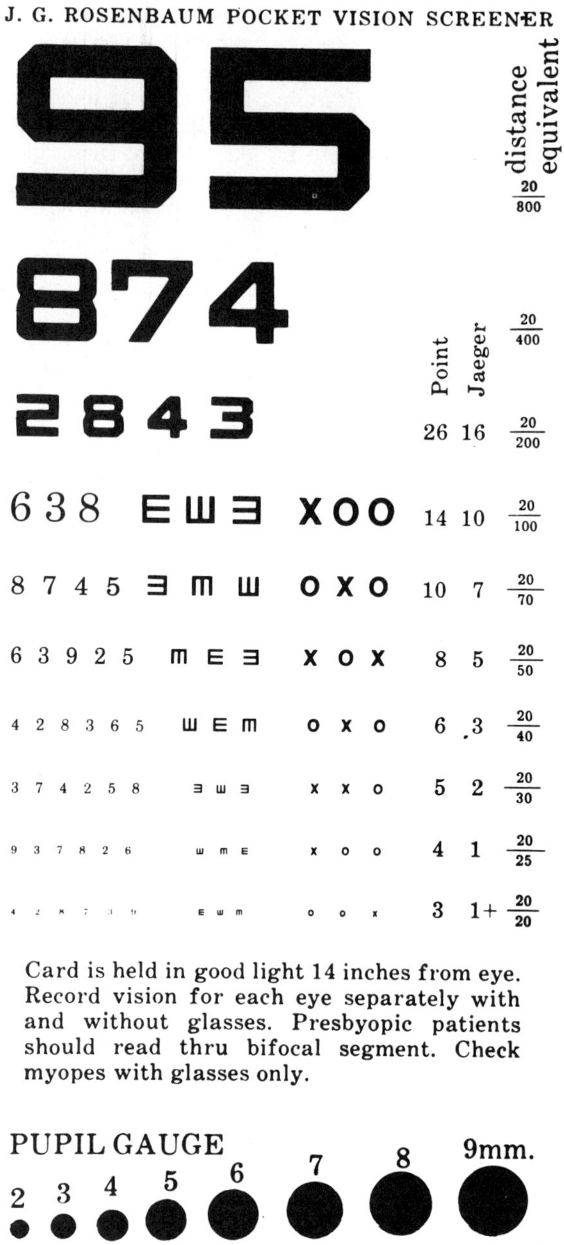

Fig. 1-3. J. G. Rosenbaum pocket vision screener.

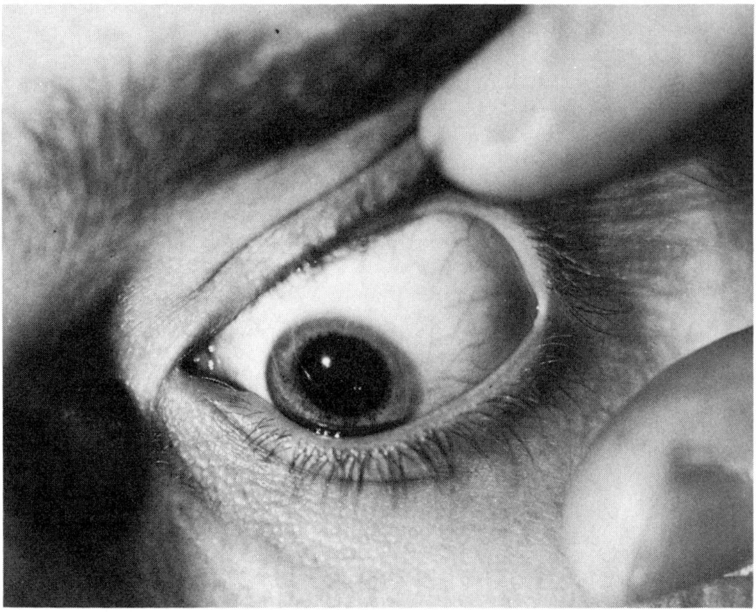

Fig. 1-4. The upper lid is elevated by pressing upward over the brow.

of the lashes may produce foreign body sensations. Abnormal closure or opening, dryness or tearing of the eye may lead the physician to different neurological disturbances or abnormalities.

When there is history of an injury in which the coats of the eye may have been lacerated, great care should be taken to avoid pressure on the eyeball. The lids may be gently palpated by sliding a finger across the closed lid surface. The upper lid can be elevated by pressing upward over the brow (Fig. 1-4). The lower lid can be inspected by pulling the skin down with a finger over the bony maxilla (Fig. 1-5).

The upper eyelid is everted easily by grasping the lashes with one hand, pulling out and down, then pressing on the lid with a thin cotton applicator stick 1 cm above the edge of the lid margin, that is, at the superior border of the tarsal plate (Figs. 1-6 A and B). The patient is requested to look down during the entire procedure. The lid should not be pushed against the

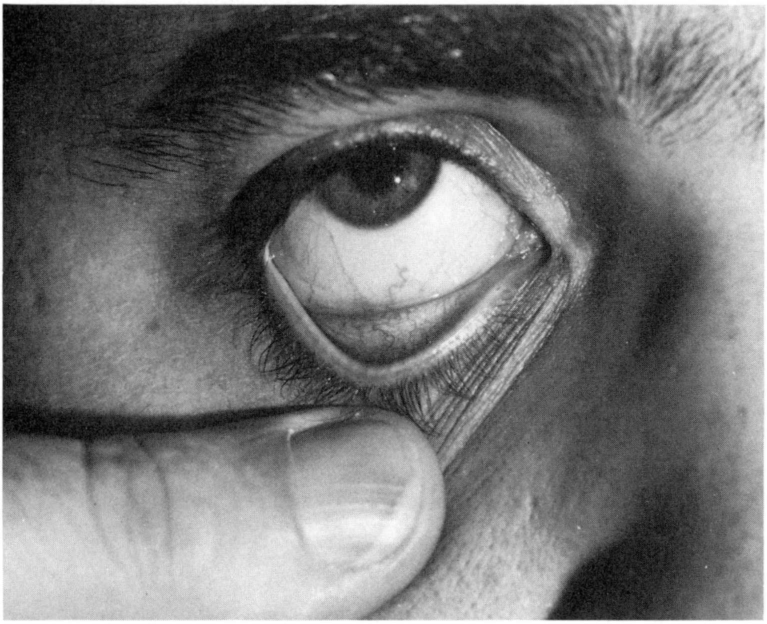

Fig. 1-5. The lower lid and conjunctival sac are inspected by pulling down the skin with a finger over the bony maxilla.

eyeball. In the presence of pain or lid spasm, it may be helpful to instill a few drops of sterile anesthetic solution in order to complete the examination properly. To restore the everted upper lid to its normal position, one should ask the patient to look up and simultaneously pull the lashes gently down.

Lacrimal Apparatus

Tears are formed in the lacrimal gland, which is situated at the superior temporal quadrant of the orbit. Part of it can be seen beneath the upper eyelid. Tears are carried from the gland to the lacrimal puncta, which is located at the nasal side of both lids. In the normal position these apertures touch the eye, the tears pass through the lacrimal canaliculi into the lacrimal sac, and from there via the nasolacrimal duct to the nose.

Examination of the normal tear flow is especially important when the patient complains about dryness or excessive tearing.

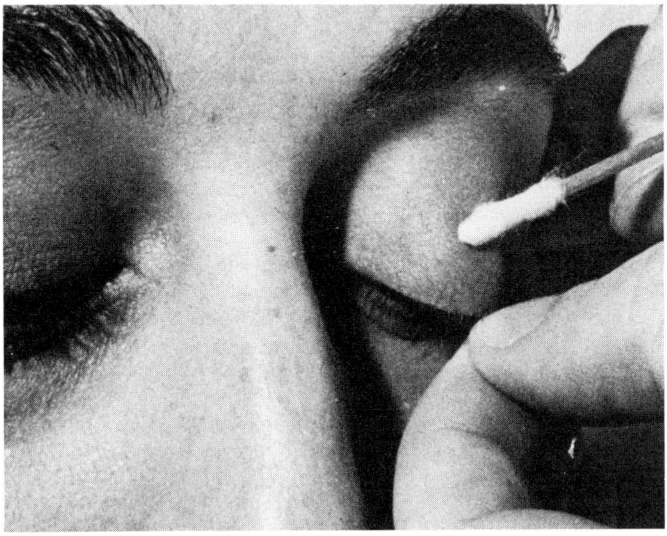

Fig. 1-6A. The upper eyelid eversion; grasp and pull down the lashes, pressing on the lid with a thin cotton applicator stick.

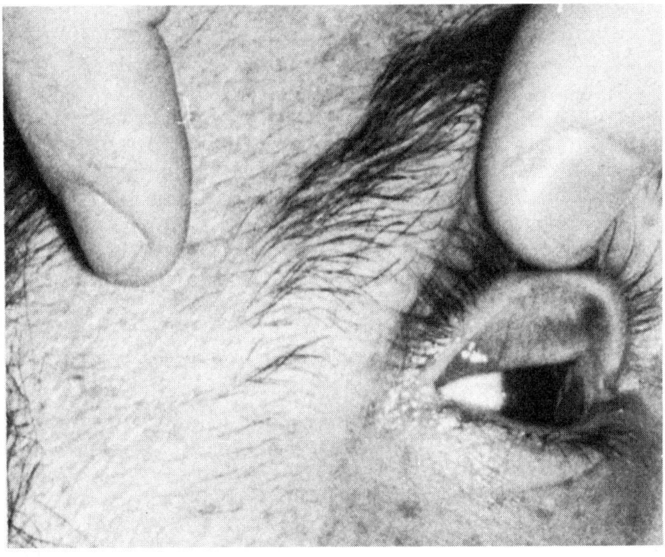

Fig. 1-6B. The everted eyelid.

In addition to determining the patency of the lacrimal puncta and the canaliculi, attention should be given to the lacrimal sac, which can be obstructed and infected. This can be examined by applying pressure on the lacrimal sac for regurgitation of infected material. The pressure is directed inside the lower inner orbital rim, not on the nose.

Conjunctiva

The palpebral conjunctiva, which lines the posterior surface of the lid, is examined at the time of lid examination. The bulbar conjunctiva is easily examined by gentle separation of the lids and having the patient look up, down, left, and right. Normal conjunctiva is almost all white and transparent. The examiner should look for injection (redness), hemorrhages, edema, foreign bodies, follicles, discolorations, secretions, and tumors. In the case of a suspected conjunctival laceration, a drop of sterile fluorescein solution might help to detect the site of the injury.

Cornea

The more sophisticated instruments to examine the cornea, such as the slit lamp, are not usually available in the emergency room. However, very often, important abnormalities of the cornea might be detected by simple external observation. Magnifying loupes can significantly aid in this examination, especially for physicians reaching the presbyopic age (Fig. 1-7). Oblique illumination with a hand lamp is often sufficient to detect the pathology of important abnormalities such as abrasion or laceration of the cornea. Abrasions of the cornea are not always visible except when stained with fluorescein. A drop of sterile fluorescein solution or a piece of filter paper saturated with fluorescein, placed in the lower cul-de-sac, helps to locate corneal abrasion or surface debris or to differentiate abrasions from corneal opacities.

Corneal sensitivity is tested by gently touching a wisp of cotton to the center of the cornea. This examination should be performed before instilling any local anesthetic. The examiner should not touch the lashes or the lids and the patient should not see the approaching cotton since this causes blinking as much as the corneal sensitivity reflex. Comparison of the corneal reflexes of both eyes is the simplest and the best standard of reference. Loss of corneal sensitivity might be the sign of local eye disease, such as dendritic ulcers (herpes simplex) or neurological abnormalities of the fifth cranial nerve.

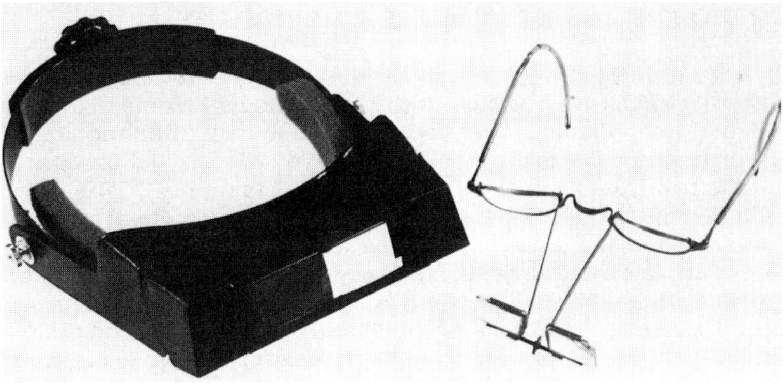

Fig. 1-7. Magnifying loupes to aid in the observation of the anterior segment.

Anterior Chamber

The depth of the anterior chamber can be determined by placing the beam of a hand light in the plane of the iris from the temporal side. If the anterior chamber is of normal depth the entire iris will be illuminated, if shallow, only the temporal half of the iris will be illuminated. The depth of the anterior chamber has important significance. The depth indicates the relative distance between the posterior surface of the cornea and the anterior iris face. In general, the anterior chamber is deep in myopes and in young persons. The chamber is usually shallow in the aged. It is in this latter group that there is concern in precipitating an acute attack of (narrow angle) glaucoma when dilating the pupil for fundus study. This acute attack is brought about by encroachment of the outflow channels of the anterior chamber angle. Whenever doubt exists about the chamber angle, gonioscopy should be performed to determine whether the chamber angle is narrow.

Iris

The iris should be noted for atrophy, changes in color, or eccentricity of the pupils. The latter may be an important sign of a perforated globe when the iris deviates into the wound.

POSITION OF THE EYES AND EYE MOVEMENTS

The size of the globe (microphthalmos = small eye, buphthalmos = large eye) and its position in the orbit should be noted. Tumor, inflammation, trauma, and thyroid disease may alter the normal position of the eyeball. When the eye has receded too much into the orbit the condition is called "enophthalmos." This could be one of the major signs of orbital floor fracture in case of a trauma to the orbit. "Exophthalmos" is the term used if the eye is displaced forward. Although abnormal displacements are recognizable by inspection, false impressions may be produced by unusual positions of the eyelid. (Widely open lids may simulate exophthalmos.) It may be necessary to take accurate measurements with an exophthalmometer.

Movements of the Extraocular Muscles

The eyes should be observed for movement together in all fields of gaze. By observing the reflection of light on the cornea one can examine the straightness of the eyes. For this purpose the easiest method is the use of a flashlight. This should be held directly in front of the patient at a distance of 1 foot. The patient is requested to look in the six cardinal positions of gaze, namely, left, right, up and right, up and left, down and right, down and left (Fig. 1-8).

Normally, the light reflection is symmetrical on both corneas. An asymmetric light reflex will betray a deviating eye.

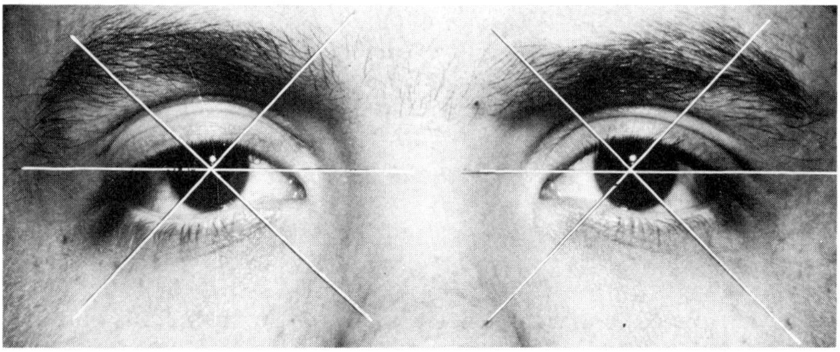

Fig. 1-8. Cardinal positions of gaze.

Location of the reflex medial to the center of the cornea indicates a divergent strabismus while location of the reflex to the temporal side indicates a convergent deviation. If the reflex is above the center, the eye is deviated downward and if the reflex is located below the center, the eye is deviated upward. An ocular deviation could be caused by a paretic or paralytic extraocular muscle. Often early signs of a neurologic abnormality can be detected by careful examination of the extraocular muscles. Double vision is a frequent complaint.

Nystagmus is an involuntary, rhythmically repeated oscillation of the eyes in any or all fields of gaze. Its importance and classification are discussed in Chapter 11.

PUPILS

The pupils should be inspected for: (1) equality, (2) size, (3) shape, and (4) reaction to stimulation (light reflex, accommodation reflex, consensual light response).

Inquiry should be made as to the use of any drug with mydriatic or miotic effect. One should never use eyedrops to dilate the pupil prior to the examination of the pupil. Normal pupils are equal in size. Unequal pupils are called "anisocoria" and may suggest previous eye disease or neurologic disorder. The term "miosis" is used when pupils are smaller than 4 mm in diameter. This can be observed in the presence of an inflammation in the anterior segment of the eye. Morphine and certain glaucoma medications cause miosis. Physiologically the pupil is miotic in sleep and in aging. The term "mydriasis" is used for enlarged pupils, that is, larger than 7 mm. The pupil is large in cases of ocular injury, systemic poisoning, and many neurologic diseases of the midbrain. Generally, the shape of the pupil is round. Irregular pupils are almost always pathologic. The shape can be affected by congenital abnormalities or by other diseases such as iritis, syphilis, or trauma.

Examination for reaction to light is best performed in a semidark room. The light should be brought from the side. The pupil contracts to direct light. Constriction of the pupil of the other eye is called "consensual pupil reaction" to light. The reaction to accommodation is tested by holding one finger or a pencil a few inches in front of the eye being tested. The patient is requested to look at the pencil and at the far wall directly beyond the pencil. The pupil constricts when looking at the near object and dilates when looking at the far object. In general, if the pupil reacts to light, it reacts to accommodation as well. An important sign of afferent defect is the Marcus-Gunn pupil. When the examiner swings a flashlight from one eye to the other, the pupil in the affected eye will dilate and fail to constrict. Argyll-Robertson pupil is a pathologic condition due to central nervous system syphilis in which there is a failure of direct and consensual light response, but a normal reaction to accommodation. Adie's pupil, or tonic pupil, responds to stimulation but very, very slowly.

MEASUREMENT OF INTRAOCULAR PRESSURE

The normal intraocular pressure is between 14 and 20 mmHg. The more common procedures used to determine intraocular pressure are: (1) finger tension, (2) measurement by Schiotz tonometer, and (3) measurement by applanation tonometer.

The simplest estimate of intraocular pressure is done by indenting the eye with the fingers (Fig. 1-9). The determination of intraocular pressure by finger is good only for gross evaluation. This type of examination should not be done in the case of a suspected lacerated eyeball.

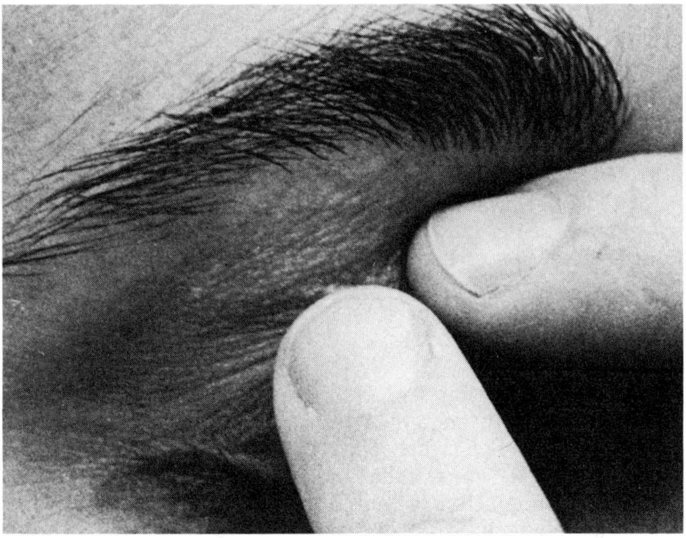

Fig. 1-9. Determination of intraocular pressure by finger technique.

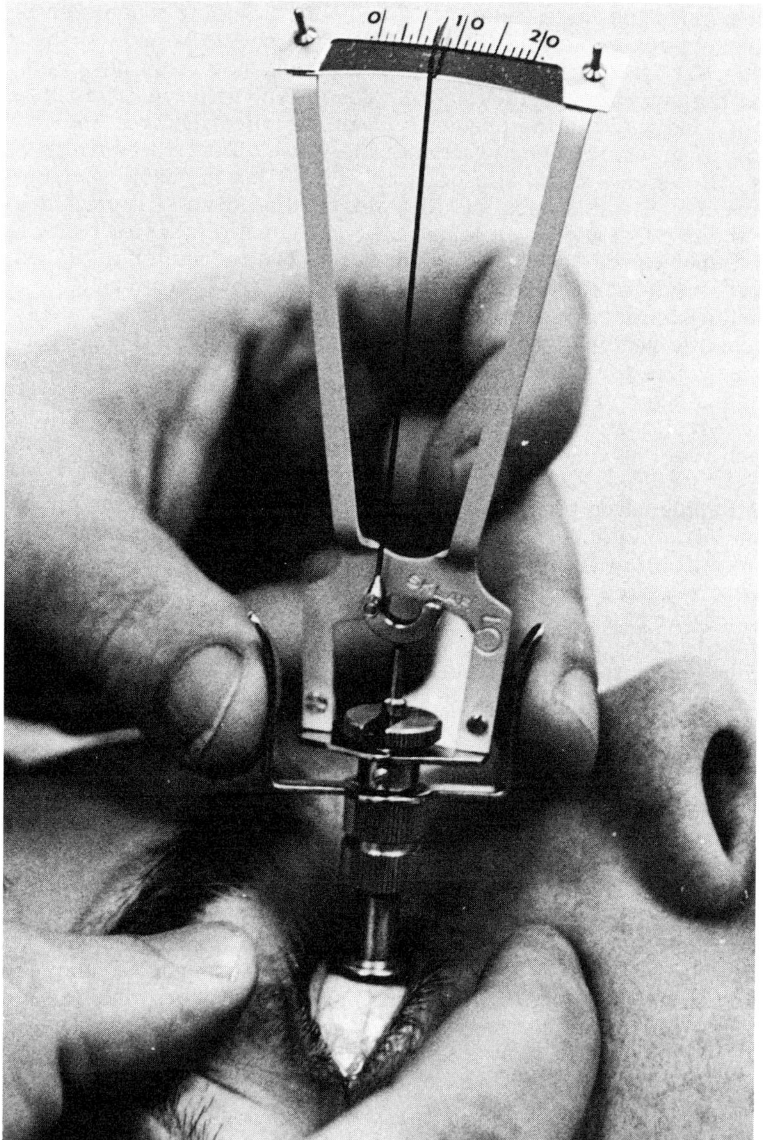

Fig. 1-10. Measurement of intraocular pressure by Schiotz tonometer.

Measuring the intraocular pressure with a Schiotz tonometer is strongly recommended (Fig. 1-10). This should be part of the general physical examination by the emergency room physician and the ophthalmologist as well. Tonometry by an instrument is contraindicated in the presence of an eye infection or in the case of an obvious perforation of the globe. The procedure is as follows: An anesthetic solution is instilled in each eye. The patient lies on his back with his shirt collar open. All pressure in the neck should be relieved. The patient is requested to look at a spot on the ceiling with both eyes. The tonometer is placed in the middle of the corneal surface of each eye. The scale reading is taken from the tonometer. A special chart converts the scale reading to mmHg. Tonometry by a Schiotz tonometer is accurate for clinical purposes in the emergency room and is adequate for primary diagnosis. To prevent spread of any ocular infection, the tonometer should be cleaned before and after each use.

The applanation tonometer is the more accurate method to measure intraocular pressure. This instrument is usually mounted on a slit lamp (Fig. 1-11). Applanation tonometry measures the force required to flatten the cornea. The end point is reached where two fluorescein semicircles are seen to slightly overlap. The pressure is read directly from the scale. This technique is more accurate than tonometry by a Schiotz tonometer.

VISUAL FIELDS

Any complete eye examination includes the visual fields. Many conditions are associated with loss of visual field. Visual fields can be examined by: (1) confrontation, (2) perimeter, and (3) tangent screen.

The confrontation test can provide useful information, especially in neurological disorders such as strokes, tumors, hemorrhages, and in some advanced ocular diseases. The technique can be made more accurate by using a white-headed pin, although a cotton-tipped applicator or pencil may be used. The patient is asked to fixate the examiner's opposite eye, i. e., right to left while the other eye is occluded. The pin is brought from the temporal side halfway between the examiner and the patient. In this way, blind spots are easily elicited and comparable. Then, the object is brought from outside the limits of the field of vision at 8-10 equally spaced meridians. Again, the field should be compared to the examiner's and should be 90° temporally, 50° nasally, 50° upward, and 65° downward (Fig. 1-12).

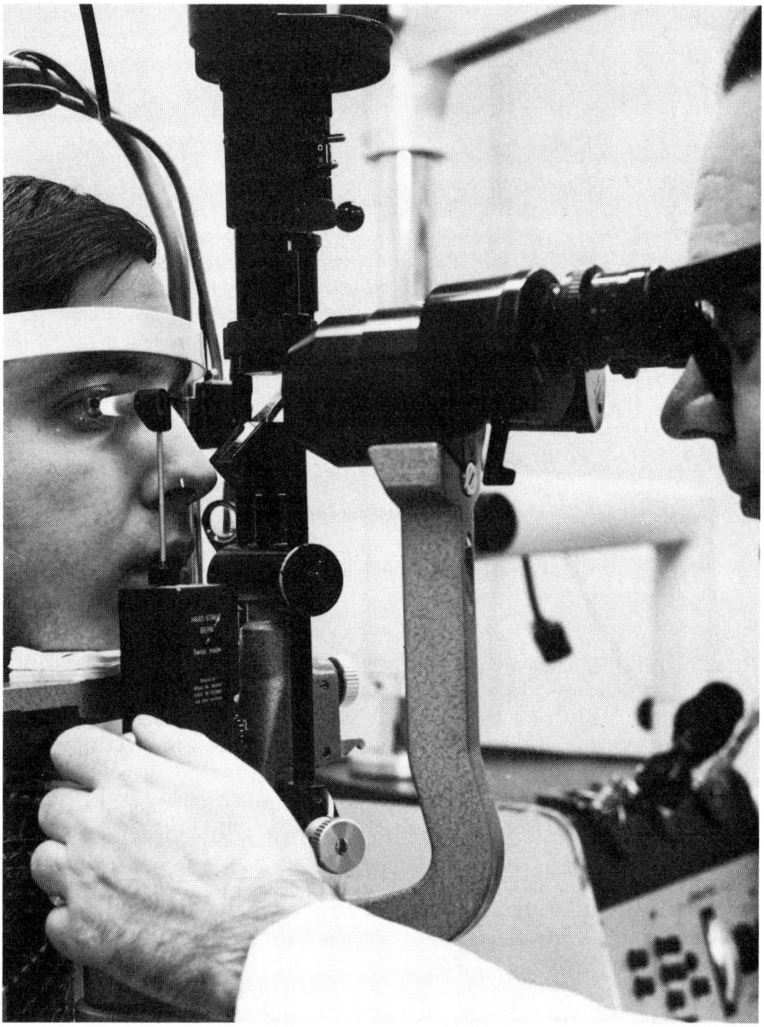

Fig. 1-11. Measurement of intraocular pressure by applanation tonometer.

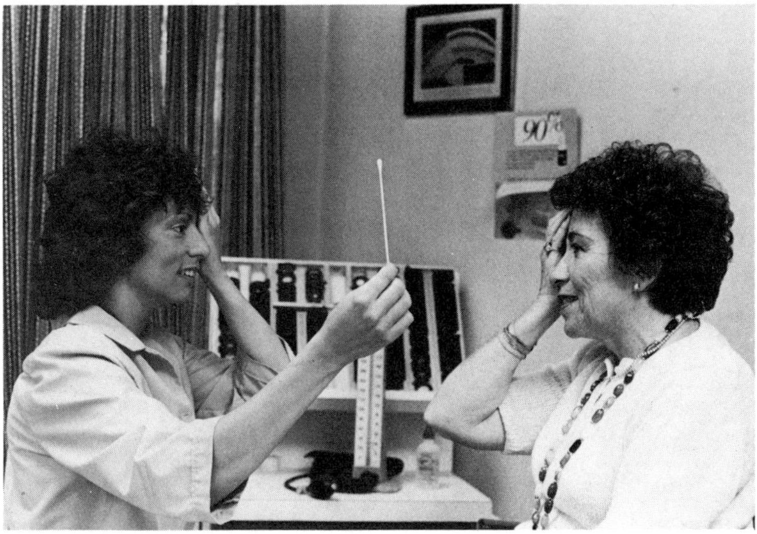

Fig. 1-12. Visual field examination by confrontation.

Several methods for accurate visual field testing are available. The tangent screen is made of black felt and is 1 meter square. It can accurately plot the central 30° field, the fixation area, and the blind spot. Various size and color test objects may be used. The auto plot, a modification of the tangent screen, allows for static testing where the object is projected to different points. This provides for more accuracy, especially when testing for glaucoma (Fig. 1-13).

With more sophisticated instruments, such as the Goldmann Perimeter (Fig. 1-14), more accuracy and better control of the patient can be obtained. There are several automated perimeters available, which have fixation monitoring devices and special programs for retesting when the patient's responses are questionable.

OPHTHALMOSCOPY

The direct ophthalmoscope is the most readily available instrument for examining the eye grounds. More sophisticated instruments, such as the indirect ophthalmoscope and special contact lenses with reflecting mirrors requiring the use of a slit lamp, are usually available only to ophthalmologists.

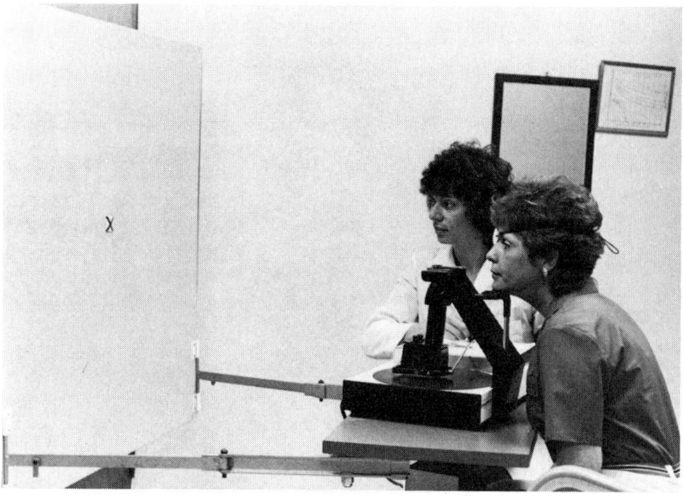

Fig. 1-13. Visual field examination by autoplot (modified tangent screen). The patient's head is on the chin rest opposite to the center of the screen.

The examination is more easily accomplished through a dilated pupil. One or two drops of Mydriacyl 1% solution (tropicamide) or Neosynephrine 2.5% is used to dilate the pupil, which greatly simplifies the examination. In the young patient, the danger of the mydriatic precipitating an attack of acute-angle closure glaucoma is negligible. In the older patient it is advisable to estimate the depth of the anterior chamber either with the direct ophthalmoscope or by means of oblique illumination. If the anterior chambers are shallow it is better not to dilate the pupils but to examine the posterior segment through the undilated pupil. The illumination in the room should be decreased. The examination requires the cooperation of the patient in that the eyes should fixate a distant object just past the examiner's ear. These rules should be observed regardless of the type of ophthalmoscope used for the examination.

Direct Ophthalmoscopy

There are many types of direct ophthalmoscopes. Source of illumination is provided either by batteries or from a wall outlet. The two main advantages of direct ophthalmoscopy are its easy handling and magnification of the picture (about 14 times).

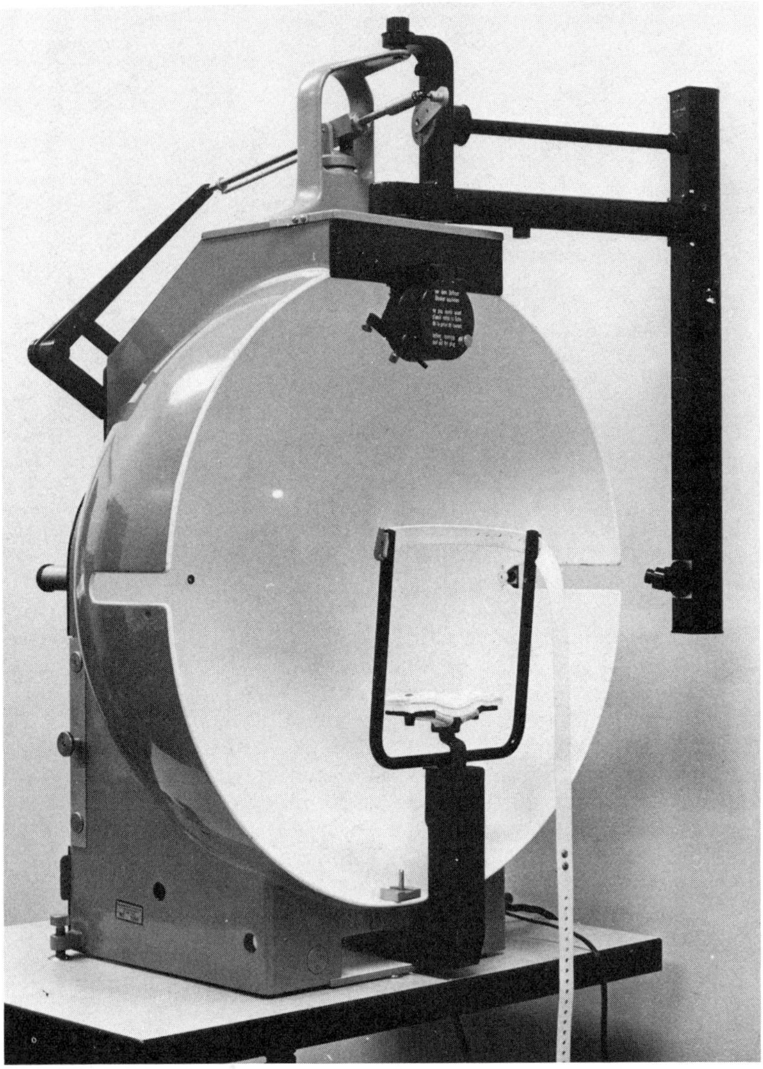

Fig. 1-14. The Goldmann Perimeter.

The ophthalmoscope should be well charged and the lenses clean. If the pupils are dilated, the larger aperture in the scope can be used but, if not dilated, the smallest aperture should be used.

The ophthalmoscope is held in the physician's right hand and in front of his right eye. When examining the patient's right eye, the physician should sit or stand at the right side of the patient (Fig. 1-15). The left hand and the left eye are used from the left side to examine the left eye.

Fundus Examination

Part A. The lens wheel is rotated to the +10 diopter lens. The light beam is directed toward the patient's pupil and the

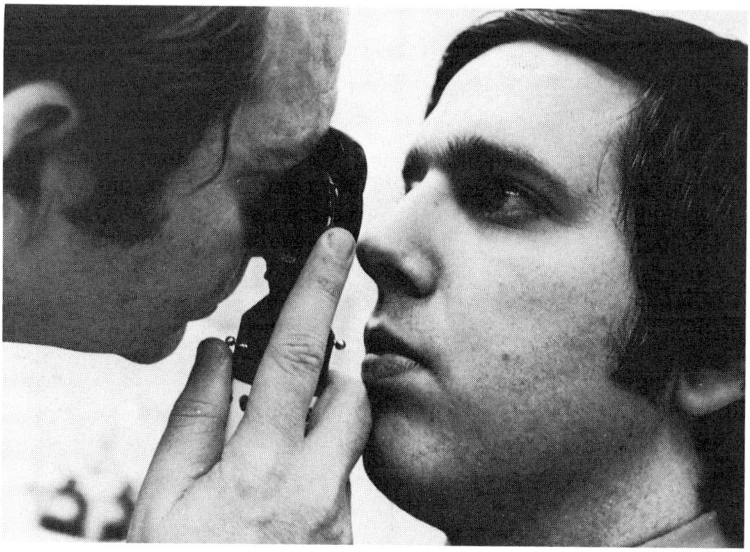

Fig. 1-15. Funduscopy using a direct ophthalmoscope. The right hand and the right eye is used from the right side to examine the right fundus.

physician brings the instrument close to the eye. First the reflex of the fundus is seen. If the eye ground is normal the reflex is red. The examiner then gradually reduces the strength of the plus lens. The focus of observation gradually progresses through the vitreous to the retina. If the lens is cataractous or the vitreous is hazy, the red reflex cannot be seen. Massive vitreous hemorrhage can cause a black fundus reflex.

Part B. If the fundus is visible, the optic disc should be examined first (Fig. 1-16). The disc can be found easily if the light is directed into the eye from a slightly temporal direction to the straight-ahead gaze of the patient.

First, the color of the disc is noted. The hyperemic disc is pink, while the atrophic disc has a grayish color. The border

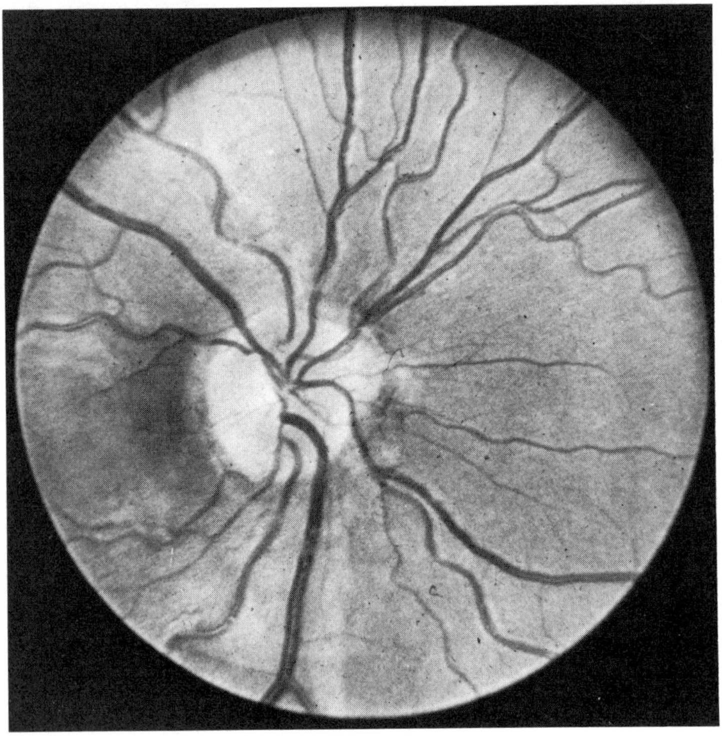

Fig. 1-16. Normal fundus appearance of the disc with the major vessels.

of the disc should be carefully examined. The normal disc has a well-defined border. Occasionally, the border of the normal disc can be blurred, primarily on the nasal side. A disc with a blurred margin usually indicates the presence of disease, especially when hemorrhages, exudates, and engorged veins are present. In the case of elevated intracranial pressure, the condition is called papilledema; in the case of an inflammatory process of the nerve head, papillitis (Fig. 1-17). The ratio between the optic cup and disc should also be noted. A large cup might be a sign of glaucoma.

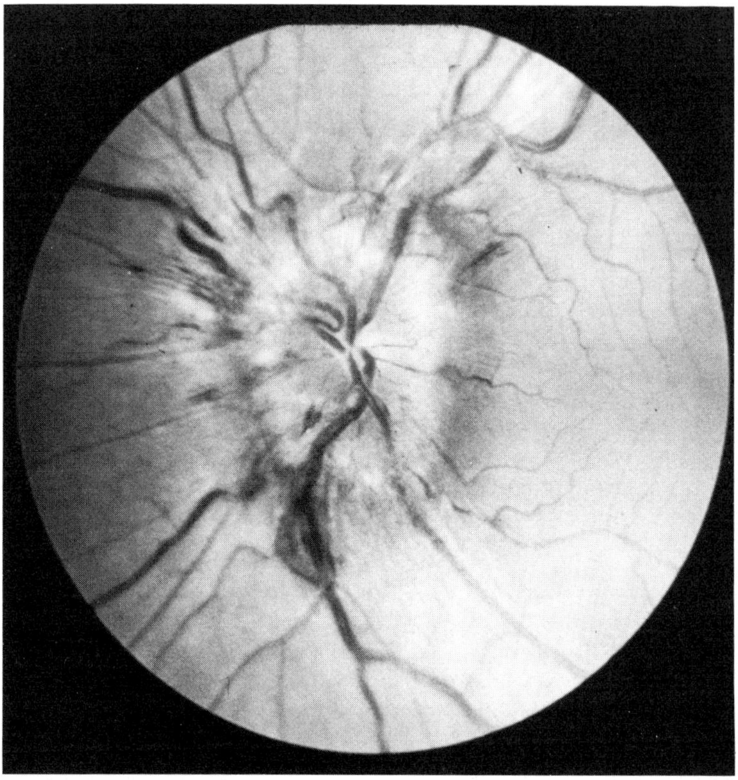

Fig. 1-17. Optic disc showing signs of papilledema: blurred disc margin, dilated veins, and hemorrhages around the disc.

Part C. The next step in the fundus examination is inspection of the vessels. The route of each main artery should be followed from the disc to the periphery, and that of each main vein from the periphery back to the disc. Narrow arteries, dilated veins, A-V compressions, hemorrhages, and exudates around the vessels should be noted. Round hemorrhages may occur in the patient with diabetes mellitus. Flame-shaped hemorrhages are a common finding in the patient with high blood pressure.

Part D. The general background of the fundus will vary with skin tones; the more pigmented the patient, the darker the fundus. Pigment clumping might be a sign of retina-choroid damage from inflammation, hemorrhages, trauma, tumors, and degenerations.

Part E. The macular area is examined in this part of the fundus examination. The easiest way is to ask the patient to look into the light of the ophthalmoscope. Normally, a red reflex of the avascular macular area is seen. In case of edema or degeneration of the retina at the macular area, the macular reflex is absent or diminished.

Part F. In the last part of the fundus examination an all-around search for pathology is performed by looking into the equatorial area and the periphery of the fundus. Fundus lesions should be located and measured. The size of a lesion is estimated by comparing it with the size of the optic disc. The size of the optic disc averages 1. 5 mm. The distance of the lesion from the disc or from the macula is recorded also. For example: The lesion is 1-disc diameter in size, is 4-disc diameters distant from the macula at the 11-o'clock position.

Indirect Ophthalmoscopy

Indirect ophthalmoscopy is used mainly by the ophthalmologist (Fig. 1-18). One advantage of this type of examination is that the illumination is stronger than that of the direct ophthalmoscope. The light may pass through opacities of the vitreous and the fundus can be visualized. A second advantage is that the fundus picture appears in three dimensions. The main disadvantage of this method is that only the well-trained ophthalmologist can perform the fundus examination with the indirect ophthalmoscope. An additional disadvantage is that the observed image is smaller than that with the direct ophthalmoscope. The magnification of the fundus is only 3 or 4 times, whereas with the direct ophthalmoscope, it is 14 times.

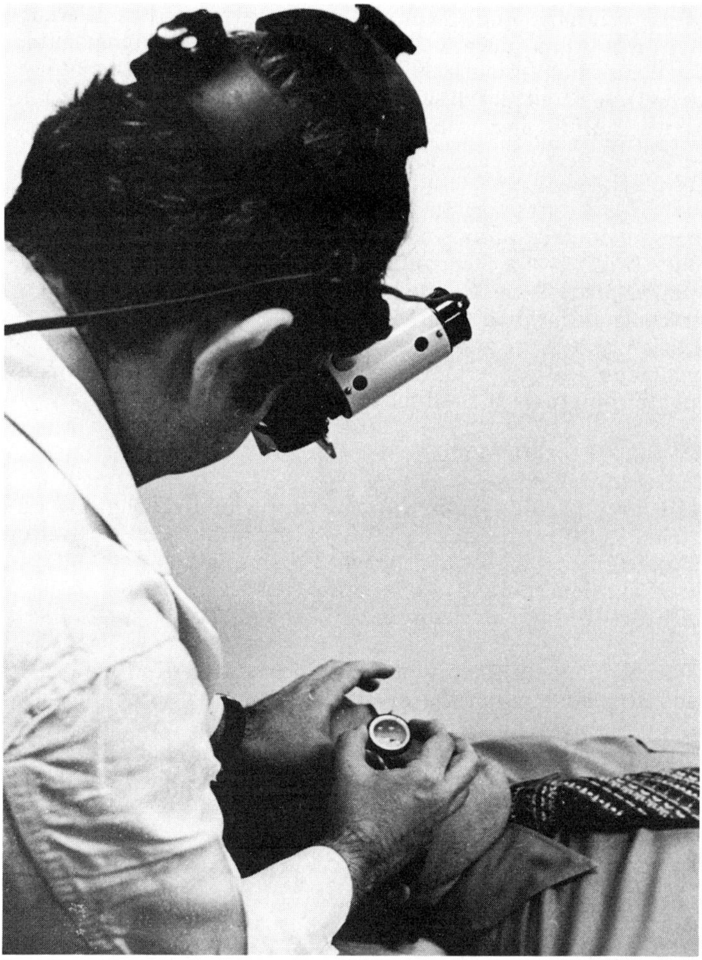

Fig. 1-18. Fundus examination by indirect ophthalmoscopy. The light source is on the head of the examiner. A 20 D lens is held in front of the eye of the patient.

SPECIAL EXAMINATIONS

The special examinations discussed in this section are not absolutely necessary to establish a diagnosis in the emergency room. However, they may provide considerable aid and can direct the ophthalmologist toward proper evaluation and treatment. In this chapter we will not mention all the sophisticated methods of eye examinations currently used in ophthalmology, but we will restrict the discussion to those methods which may actually be helpful in an emergency situation.

CONTACT LENS EXAMINATION

The contact lens examination is reserved for the ophthalmologist only (Fig. 1-19). Therefore, it is mentioned only briefly. The examination is performed with the aid of a slit lamp. A contact lens with three mirrors is placed on the cornea after instillation of a local anesthetic solution. This type of examination provides a highly magnified, well-illuminated, and three-dimensional picture of the fundus.

SLIT-LAMP EXAMINATION

The slit lamp is a binocular microscope with a strong source of light (Fig. 1-20). It provides a highly magnified and well-illuminated view of the area which might be involved in disease or trauma. The instrument is especially useful when one suspects a small foreign body or laceration of the cornea.

The patient places his chin on the chin rest and his forehead presses slightly against the plastic frame. The ophthalmologist examines the eyes by moving the instrument into focus with a small handle situated on the table of the instrument. The lids and the anterior segment of the eye can be examined easily. If

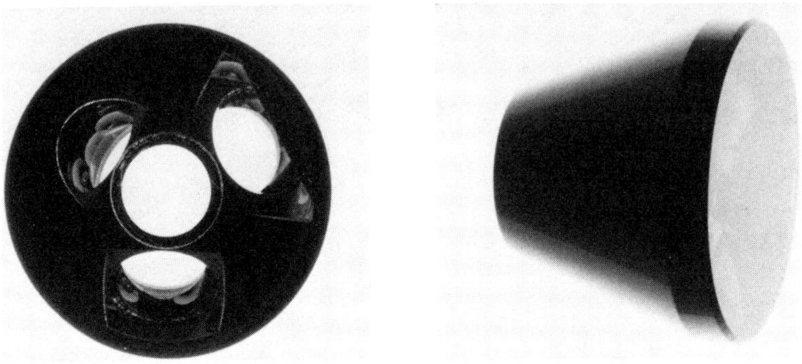

Fig. 1-19. Goldmann three-mirror contact lens.

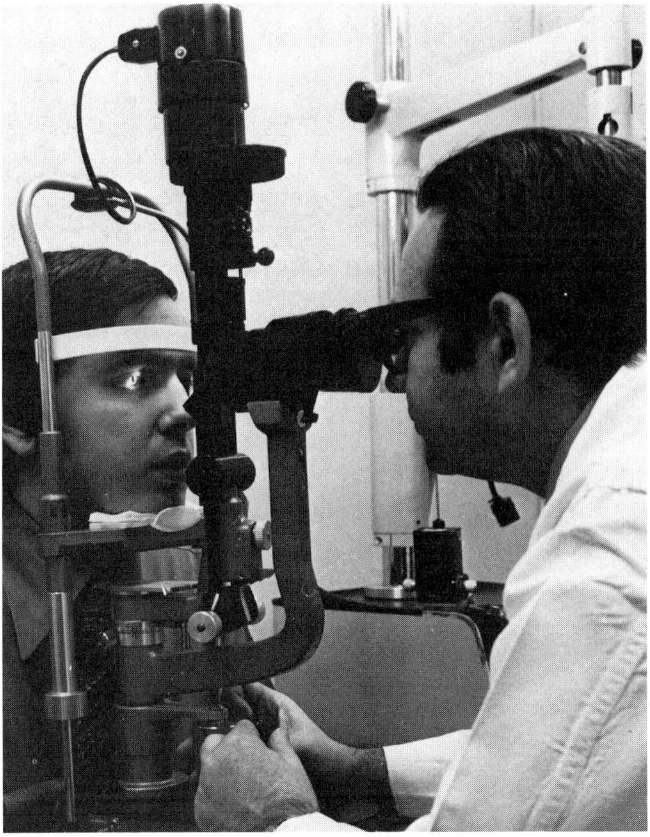

Fig. 1-20. Slit-lamp examination.

the pupil is dilated, the lens is checked for opacities or dislocation. To examine the posterior segment of the eye, a contact lens is placed on the cornea.

EXOPHTHALMOMETRY

Although abnormal prominence or backward displacement of the eye is recognizable by inspection, proper measurements may be taken with the exophthalmometer (Fig. 1-21). With this instrument, one can measure the anteroposterior distance between the most anterior part of the cornea and the lateral orbital rim. The exophthalmometer is placed against the bony

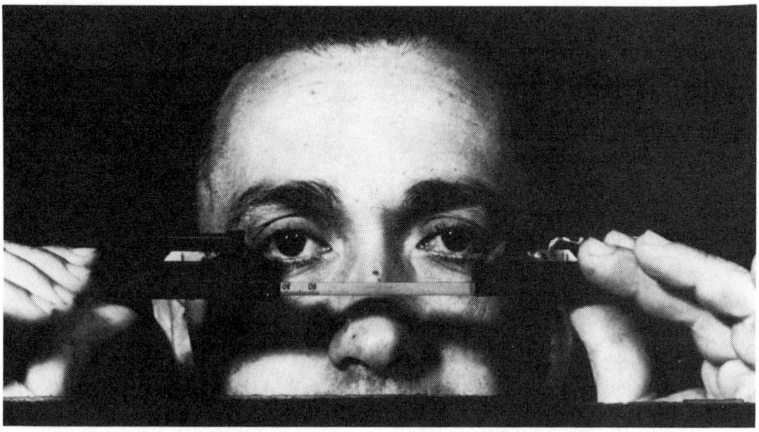

Fig. 1-21. Exophthalmometry. The exophthalmometer measures the anteroposterior distance between the most anterior part of the cornea and the bony lateral orbital rim.

orbital margin on both sides and the bar reading is noted. This number is the distance in millimeters between the two bony orbital walls. The physician then views the corneas in the instrument's mirror. The corneas are simultaneously lined up with a scale in millimeters. The measurements are noted again. Both the bar reading and the protrusion of the eyes are recorded. Example: 98-19/18 means that the bar reading is 98 mm; right eye protrudes 19 mm; left eye, 18 mm. For successive comparative measurements, the bar reading of the same patient should always be the same. Normal range of protrusion of the eyes averages between 12 and 20 mm. Exophthalmic measurements are over 21 mm (Fig. 1-22). If there is no protrusion, both eyes should give equal or almost equal measurements.

X-RAY, ULTRASOUND CAT SCAN

These examinations of the eye and orbit are discussed in a separate chapter.

BACTERIOLOGIC EXAMINATION

Bacteriologic examinations are indicated in cases of external infection with secretion, or in suspected intraocular infection before starting any treatment. The procedure is divided into

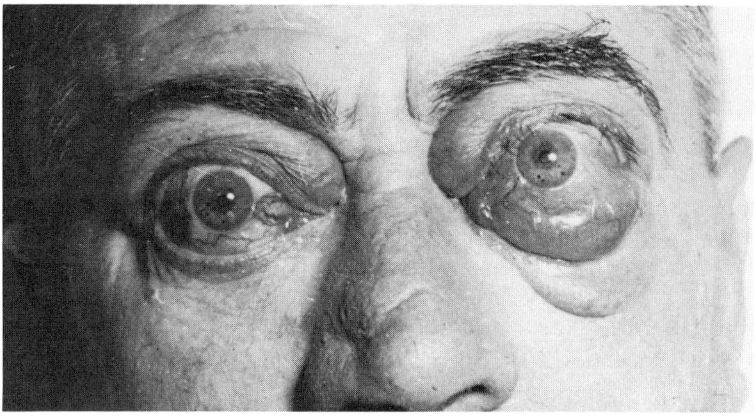

Fig. 1-22. Bilateral exophthalmos and chemosis. The right eye protrudes 25 mm, the left eye protrudes 26 mm.

two parts. First, the suspected area (corneal ulcer) is scraped with a sterile spatula or secretion material is removed from the lower cul-de-sac and smeared on a glass slide. After this material is dried, the smear is stained with one of the commonly available stains (Gram, Giemsa, KOH). The smear is then studied under the microscope. Bacteria or hyphae of fungus, eosinophils, or other white cells can be identified in this manner. The second part of the examination consists of taking culture samples from the infected area and from the cul-de-sac for incubation in different culture media. This part of the examination can be very helpful if the initial treatment proved to be ineffective and a change in treatment is indicated, based on the findings of the cultures.

BIBLIOGRAPHY

Collins, J.: Handbook of Clinical Ophthalmology. Masson Publishers, NY, 1982.

Gittinger, J.: Ophthalmology. A Clinical Introduction. Little, Brown and Company, Boston, 1984.

Kupfer, C. and Kaiser, M.: Disorders of the Eye and Visual Systems. Differential Diagnosis. ARCO Diagnostic Series, 1978.

Newell, F. W.: Ophthalmology Principles and Concepts, 5th ed. Mosby, St. Louis, 1982.

Chapter 2

SUDDEN LOSS OR DETERIORATION OF VISION

When a patient presents with a sudden loss of vision, the physician must quickly assess whether this is an ophthalmologic emergency which demands immediate and complete attention or whether the situation can be treated at a slightly later time. A brief ocular history should be obtained which should concentrate on whether or not the patient has a total loss of vision, whether it was gradual or sudden, if associated with pain, and whether there were any associated signs and symptoms, such as flashing lights and loss of peripheral vision. One must next check the patient's vision and then immediately check for an afferent pupillary defect (APD). An afferent pupillary defect is defined as an asymmetry of the pupillary response to light in each eye. The range of this defect can be from trace to 4+ (an amaurotic eye). When a pupil, which constricted when the opposite eye was exposed to light, dilates when light is shined into it, it is known as a Marcus-Gunn pupil. For the purposes in this chapter, when the term "afferent pupillary defect" is used, it will refer to a Marcus-Gunn pupil.

If an afferent pupillary defect is not found, the situation usually does not demand immediate and complete attention. However, should an afferent pupillary defect be present, then one must, even through an undilated pupil, quickly assess the retina. If the retina and optic nerve both appear normal, the presumed diagnosis must be a central retinal artery occlusion. This patient then must receive immediate attention and all other concerns must be put aside. Since the most common cause of a central artery occlusion is an embolism, the immediate treatment should include ocular massage, rebreathing into a brown paper bag, and determining whether or not to perform an anterior chamber paracentesis. In older patients, a tube of blood should be drawn for an ESR to rule out temporal arteritis.

The presence of an afferent pupillary defect suggests the following etiologies: central retinal artery occlusion, central retinal vein occlusion, or optic neuritis.

In the absence of an afferent pupillary defect, one should consider the following etiologies: (1) retinal detachment, (2) degenerative maculopathy, (3) inflammatory maculopathy, (4) hemorrhagic maculopathy, (5) vitreous hemorrhage, (6) acute glaucoma, (7) trauma, (8) hysteria, and (9) poisoning.

SUDDEN VISUAL LOSS WITH AFFERENT PUPILLARY DEFECT

CENTRAL RETINAL ARTERY OCCLUSION

If a patient presents within 100 minutes of a central retinal artery occlusion, there is a possibility of returning that eye to normal vision. Initially an embolus should be considered and measures must be taken to cause dilation of the central retinal artery in the hope that the embolus will pass distally.

While the most common etiology for an artery occlusion is an atheromatous plaque, emboli arising from the major vessels, the valves of the heart, the chambers of the heart, or simply from platelet aggregation may be responsible (Fig. 2-1). It should be noted that in an older individual one must always rule out temporal arteritis. This can be done by obtaining a stat ESR as well as palpating the temporal arteries. However, the key point, which must be restated, is that for an eye with a sudden loss of vision, an afferent pupillary defect, and a normal appearing fundus, the presumed diagnosis must be a central retinal artery occlusion.

Signs and Symptoms

There is a sudden, painless deterioration of vision in the affected eye. Visual acuity can be reduced to light perception or complete blindness. The pupil does not react or reacts sluggishly to direct light stimulus. On fundus examination the disc

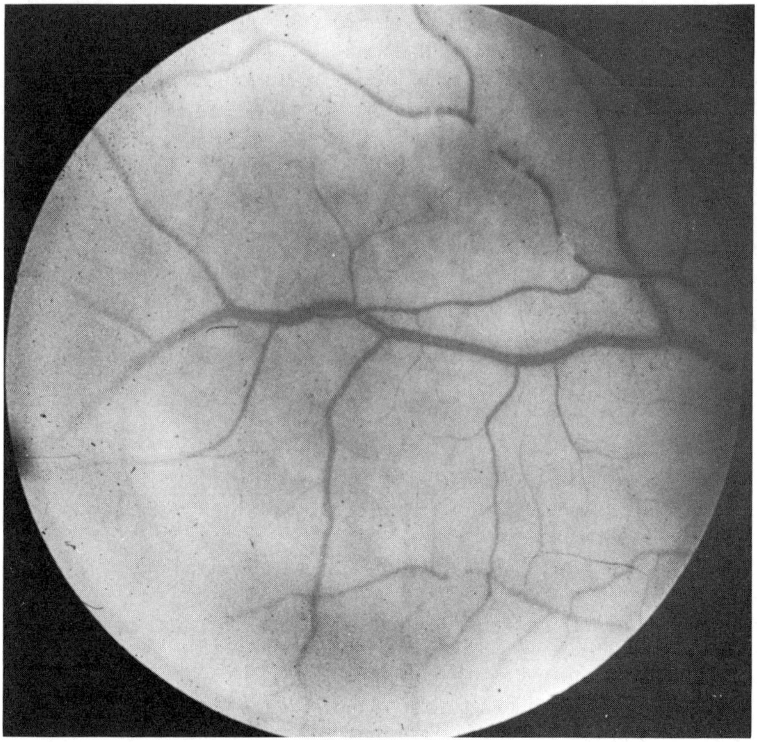

Fig. 2-1. Multiple emboli in the upper temporal retinal artery. Medical investigation proved that the emboli originated from an eroded atheromatous plaque in the common carotid artery.

is pale and the veins appear dark. The arterioles are narrowed and less frequently show sludging. After the early stages of the occlusion, there is marked edema of the retina corresponding to the occluded artery. If the central retinal artery is occluded, the whole posterior pole is edematous and, except for the fovea, appears whitish (Fig. 2-2). The foveal area transmits its normal red choroidal color, because at the fovea the retina is thin. No ganglion cells are present. This is known as the "cherry red" spot, a sign of occlusion of the central retinal artery. In branch occlusion the pallor of the fundus is confined to the area supplied by the affected artery (Fig. 2-3).

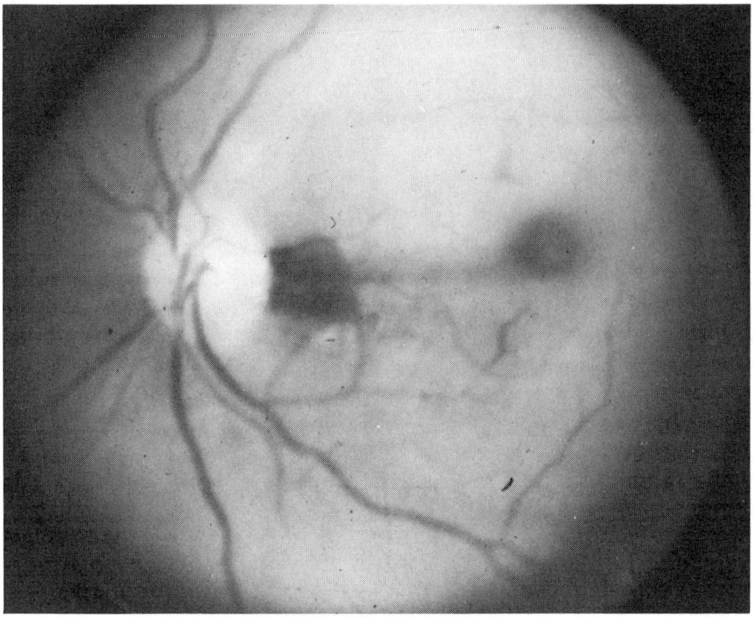

Fig. 2-2. Retinal artery occlusion. The foveal area appears dark when compared to the surrounding retina, which is pale and edematous.

Treatment

The patient must receive a breathing bag and ocular massage. An assessment of the risk/benefit ratio for an anterior chamber tap must be considered. If the artery occlusion is more than 100 minutes old and the retina is already white, it is doubtful that vision can be restored. However, the patient should still receive treatment.

Before sending the patient for a thorough medical evaluation, one should consider treatment with aspirin (1 tab b. i. d. until workup has been done). This may, of course, invalidate platelet studies, but it may also prevent platelet emboli from going to other areas of the central nervous system. With aspirin therapy, the risk/benefit ratio of treatment should be assessed.

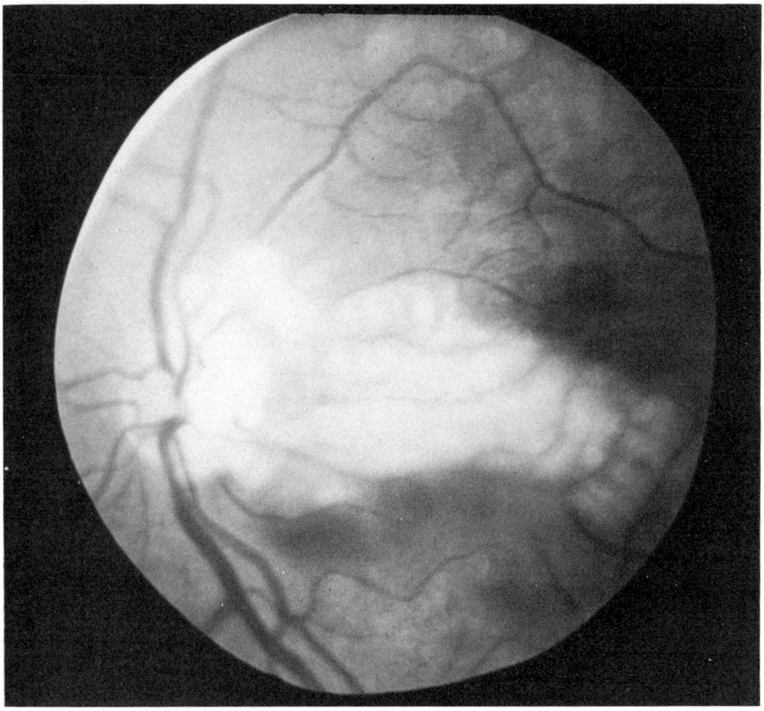

Fig. 2-3. Branch occlusion of the retinal artery. The pallor is confined to the area served by the affected artery.

CENTRAL RETINAL VEIN OCCLUSION

Central retinal vein occlusion can occur in almost any age range, but it is most common in older patients with either glaucoma, diabetes, or hypertension. Central vein occlusions should be considered as either venous stasis retinopathy or hemorrhagic (ischemic) retinopathy. That breakdown is considered crucial to prognosis. Most cases of venous stasis retinopathy require no treatment and do rather well. Vision may drop to the 20/200 level or lower, but often the patient maintains relatively good vision. Patients with ischemic or hemorrhagic central retinal vein occlusion, however, rarely retain good vision. Fluorescein angiography of these cases may show massive capillary dropout. There is currently some controversy as to the best mode of treatment. Some believe that if pressure on the eye elicits venous pulsation, then the patient cannot have had a complete occlusion of the central retinal vein and, therefore, rubeosis and neovascular glaucoma are not possible. If, however, spontaneous venous pulsations cannot be elicited and instead one obtains arterial pulsations, then the retinal vein has been totally occluded, and there is a chance that this patient may develop rubeosis iridis and neovascular glaucoma. Others, however, prefer to do fluorescein angiography and total the amount of nonperfused tissue. If the amount of capillary nonperfusion is significant, then prophylactic panretinal photocoagulation is recommended. The underlying problem is that approximately 30% of patients with central retinal vein occlusions develop neovascular glaucoma in approximately 3 months. This is referred to as "90-day glaucoma," a severe and intractable disease. If one considers only ischemic central retinal vein occlusions, the percentage of patients who develop rubeosis iridis and neovascular glaucoma is significantly greater than 30%.

The workup of the patient with central retinal vein occlusion is often disappointing. Polycythemia, leukemia, macroglobulinemia, and cryoglobulinemia are several hematological disorders which can predispose or cause a central retinal vein occlusion. Additionally, some young, healthy adults can develop central retinal vein occlusions thought to be associated with birth control pills, pregnancy, reduced systemic blood pressure, increased orbital or intraocular pressure, pressure on the veins or optic nerve, or any inflammation which could cause closure of the vein.

Signs and Symptoms

Sudden or gradual painless severe deterioration of visual acuity occurs in central vein occlusions. Visual acuity may be reduced to a minimal amount or to a great amount, such as hand movements, light perception only, or no light perception.

Examination of the fundus ranges from mild to moderate tortuosity of the retinal veins to the "blood and thunder" retinopathy of an ischemic central retinal vein occlusion. The anterior segment of the eye shows little involvement. Occasionally, the vessels in the iris are dilated and engorged. In the typical ophthalmoscopic picture of the central retinal vein occlusion, the optic disc is deep red and its border is blurred because of swelling.

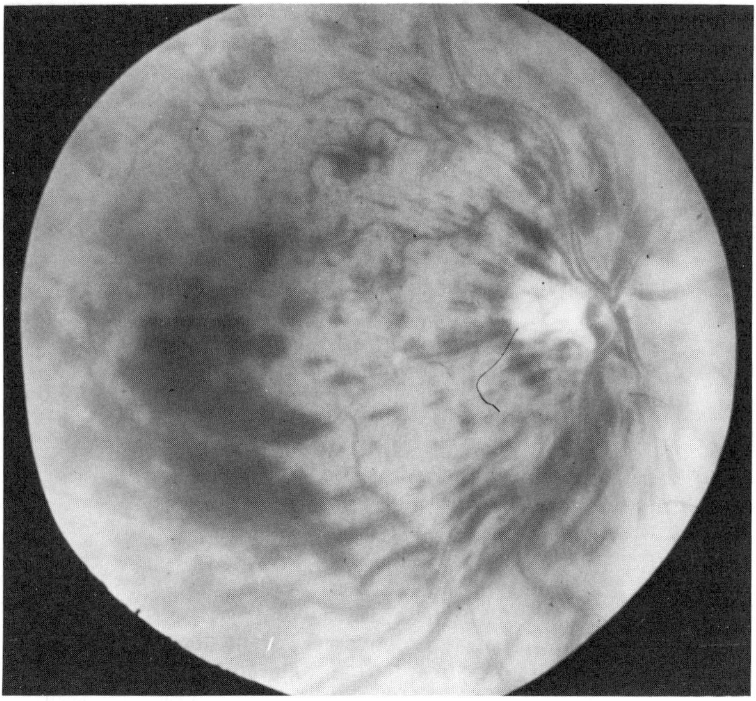

Fig. 2-4. Central retinal vein occlusion. The border of the optic disc is hardly seen. Multiple hemorrhages of different size and shape are seen all around the posterior pole. The veins are considerably engorged.

Multiple hemorrhages are seen all around the optic disc, and the posterior pole and may extend far into the periphery. The size and shape of the hemorrhages are variable. The hemorrhages may be small or large, flame-shaped, or round. They may be superficial or deep. The arteries are narrow. The veins are engorged and their color is much darker than in the normal fundus. Cotton wool patches, when present, are more frequent around the optic disc (Fig. 2-4).

The ophthalmoscopic appearance of the branch occlusion is

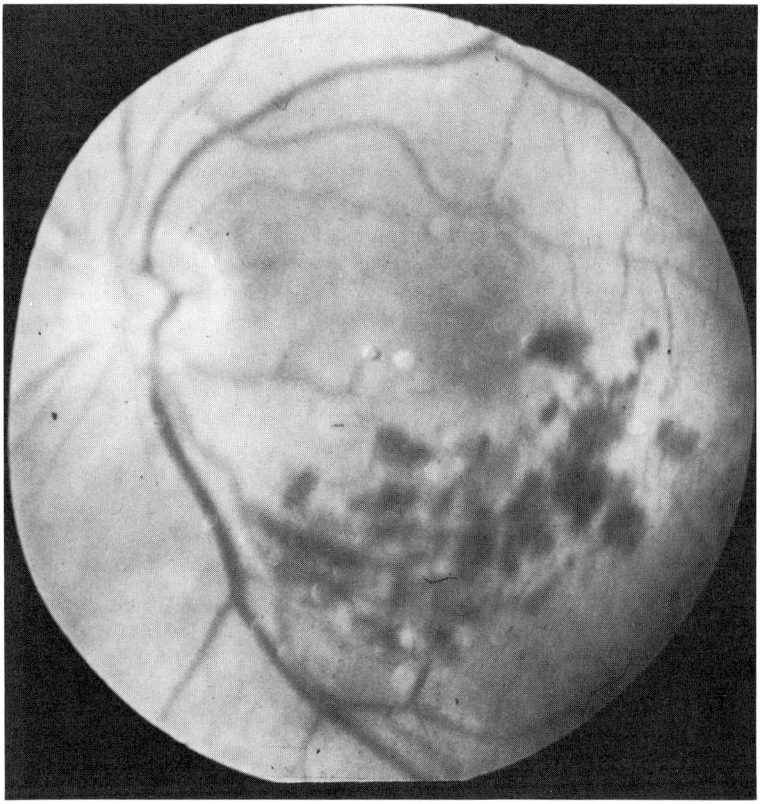

Fig. 2-5. Branch occlusion of the central retinal vein. Hemorrhages are seen along the occluded vessel.

much less dramatic. The optic disc is not involved. Hemorrhages, exudates, and vascular changes can be seen all around the occluded vein. As in the case of central retinal vein occlusion, the size and shape of the hemorrhages and exudates are variable (Fig. 2-5).

Differential Diagnosis

Central vein occlusion is a unilateral disease. Ophthalmoscopic appearance is similar to that of diabetic retinopathy, which is a bilateral disease that causes gradual rather than sudden changes in vision. The same is true in the case of severe hypertension; both eyes are involved almost equally and the vision is relatively good.

When branch vein occlusion is diagnosed, vasculitis must be considered in the differential diagnosis.

As the central retinal vein occlusion clears, collateral veins can be seen on the disc which have been inappropriately called "optociliary shunt vessels." These are actually collateral vessels and not shunts. These are also seen with optic nerve tumors, chronic papilledema, and even in some patients with glaucoma. They remain even after the patient's "blood and thunder" retinopathy has resolved.

OPTIC NEURITIS

See Chapter 11.

SUDDEN VISUAL LOSS WITHOUT AFFERENT PUPILLARY DEFECTS

RETINAL DETACHMENTS

Retinal detachments are of three types: exudative, tractional, and rhegmatogenous. By far, the most common of the three are rhegmatogenous detachments, which are caused by vitreoretinal traction producing a tear in the retina through which fluid passes and causes the neurosensory retina to detach from the pigment epithelium (Fig. 2-6). The patient may commonly have a history of eye trauma, aphakia, or myopia. When the macula detaches, the patient loses central vision. When there is a rhegmatogenous retinal detachment and the macula is still attached, the condition is a surgical emergency. Upon examination with the indirect ophthalmoscope, an acute retinal detachment shows retinal edema and the retina appears rather grey.

Signs and Symptoms

The patient may complain of floaters resulting from blood or pigment epithelial cells or flashes of light from vitreoretinal traction. The patient may complain of a shadow or curtain which obscures a portion of the visual field. If the detachment does not involve the macula, visual acuity may remain normal. A severe loss in central vision occurs when the macula area is detached. Often, the patient does not consider seriously the

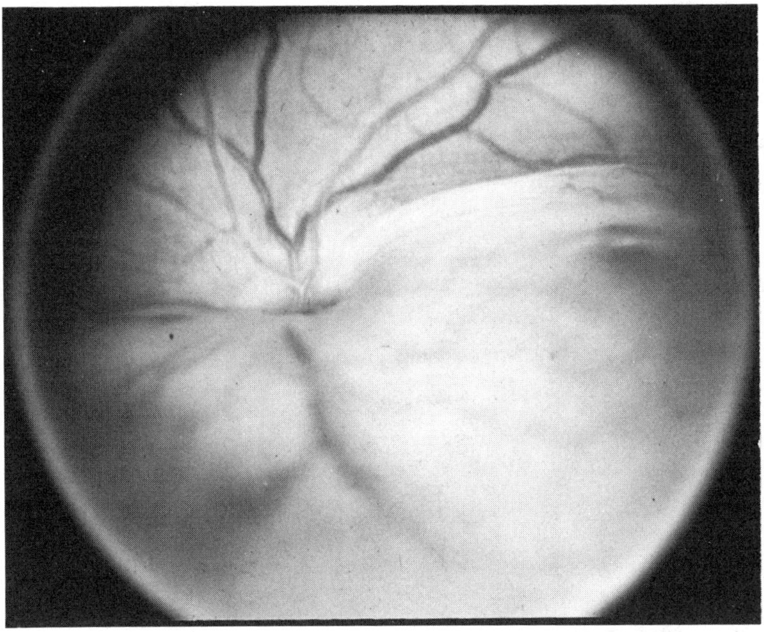

Fig. 2-6. Bullous retinal detachment. The lower half of the retina is detached.

signs of peripheral retinal detachment, namely seeing a shadow, and comes to the emergency room because of sudden deterioration of vision when detachment of the macula occurs. The visual acuity is then usually reduced to hand motion. In most cases the intraocular pressure remains normal or slightly below normal. The freshly detached retina looks grey, occasionally with white folds in it and may have a globular, bullous appearance. In a rhegmatogenous detachment, retinal holes or tears are present. Holes may be horseshoe-shaped or round. In most cases the holes occur at the equatorial area or anterior to it. To view retinal breaks one must use the indirect ophthalmoscope.

Treatment

The surgical goal of treating a rhegmatogenous retinal detachment is to find all the retinal tears and close them. This is commonly done with cryopexy or diathermy; then the retina is supported with a scleral buckle. If one cannot find the retinal tear, an exudative detachment secondary to a tumor, inflammatory process, or a vascular lesion should be ruled out.

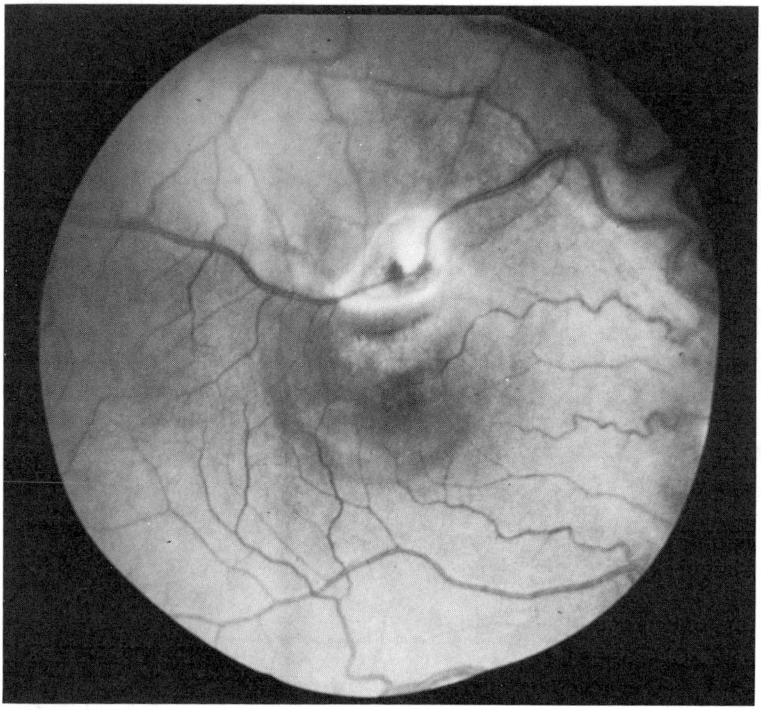

Fig. 2-7. Subretinal neovascular membrane in the macula. The vision was 20/400.

DEGENERATIVE MACULOPATHY

The most common form of this condition is seen with macular degeneration of aging, unfortunately known as senile macular degeneration. These patients develop excrescences in Bruch's membrane (drusen). This may lead to geographic atrophy of the retinal pigment epithelium (RPE) or focal RPE detachments. Any time there is a defect in the RPE, blood vessels may emerge from the choroid and grow into the subretinal space (Fig. 2-7). This can then become a "disciform" scar.

Signs and Symptoms

If geographic areas of atrophy of the RPE develop, the patient generally has a gradual loss of vision. Detachments of the RPE or hemorrhages from subretinal neovascular membranes can cause a sudden loss of vision. All of these visual changes are completely painless.

Treatment

Subretinal neovascular membranes can be treated with the Argon laser if the membrane lies outside the capillary free zone (CFZ). If the membrane grows into the CFZ but does not completely underlie it, treatment may be possible with the Argon green or Krypton laser. It is very important to obtain stereoscopic fluorescein angiograms before attempting to treat these membranes. It is important to realize that these membranes can recur after treatment and that very few of the patients with macular degeneration are treatable with any laser.

INFLAMMATORY MACULOPATHY

These inflammatory changes are most commonly endogenous. The most frequent causes are toxoplasmosis, septic emboli (usually from endocarditis), autoimmune disease, or viral infections. There are other inflammatory causes for which the etiology is unknown, such as serpiginous choroiditis, acute multifocal posterior placquoid pigment epitheliopathy (AMPPPE), and acute retinal pigment epithelialitis (ARPE). With all of these conditions, vitritis is present but the anterior chamber is usually free of cells.

Signs and Symptoms

The patient complains of loss of vision if the fovea is involved. If the fovea is not involved, the patient may complain only of floaters. The patient will complain of pain only if there is a cellular reaction in the anterior chamber.

Treatment

In addition to deterioration of vision, the autoimmune conditions require only steroid treatment. Endogenous endophthalmitis requires treatment of the primary infection as well as intravitreal antibiotics. Serpiginous choroiditis, AMPPPE, and ARPE are all conditions which have no known treatment. Before treating any patient with steroids, there should be no medical contraindication to their use. Conditions such as tuberculosis, peptic ulcer, diabetes, and hypertension are all problems which the treating physician must be prepared to deal with. Topical treatment, such as cycloplegics and topical steroids, are necessary only if there is anterior chamber involvement. Topical medications go no further than the anterior third of the vitreous in the phakic eye. Treatment depends on the diagnosis. The patient with toxoplasmosis is given triple sulfa, folinic acid, and prednisone if central vision is threatened. Some centers now recommend oral clindamycin and prednisone. In either case, it is obvious that one is treating both the Toxoplasma organism and the inflammation.

HEMORRHAGIC MACULOPATHY

Macular hemorrhages usually cause an abrupt loss of vision. These can occur with vascular tissue under the retina or from vascular problems within the retina. Vascular membranes under the retina most often occur with macular degeneration of aging (covered under Degenerative Maculopathy) but can also occur with high myopia, trauma, or chorioretinitis (Fig. 2-8). The pathophysiology of all these conditions involves defects in the RPE through which subretinal neovascular membranes can grow.

Vascular problems within the retina can also cause a sudden loss of vision. These problems can be seen in systemic diseases, such as leukemia, anemia, thrombocytopenia, diabetes mellitus, or hypertension. Macular hemorrhages can also occur secondary to a Valsalva maneuver, retinal telangiectasia, and branch retinal vein occlusion or secondary to increased intracapillary pressure. A branch retinal artery occlusion causes a sudden loss of vision but presents with a pale, infarcted retina rather than a hyperemic retina.

Signs and Symptoms

The patient complains of an abrupt, painless loss of vision. If the hemorrhage lies under the retina and has drusen associated with it, then this is most likely due to a subretinal neovascular membrane lying either immediately under the retina or the RPE. This is described under Degenerative Maculopathy.

If the hemorrhages lie within the retina, then one must decide if it represents a branch retinal vein occlusion, retinal telangiectasia, or perhaps some systemic disease such as diabetes. Hemorrhages that lie under the internal limiting lamina and on the nerve fiber layer are called "preretinal hemorrhages" and often layer out secondary to gravity. These are termed

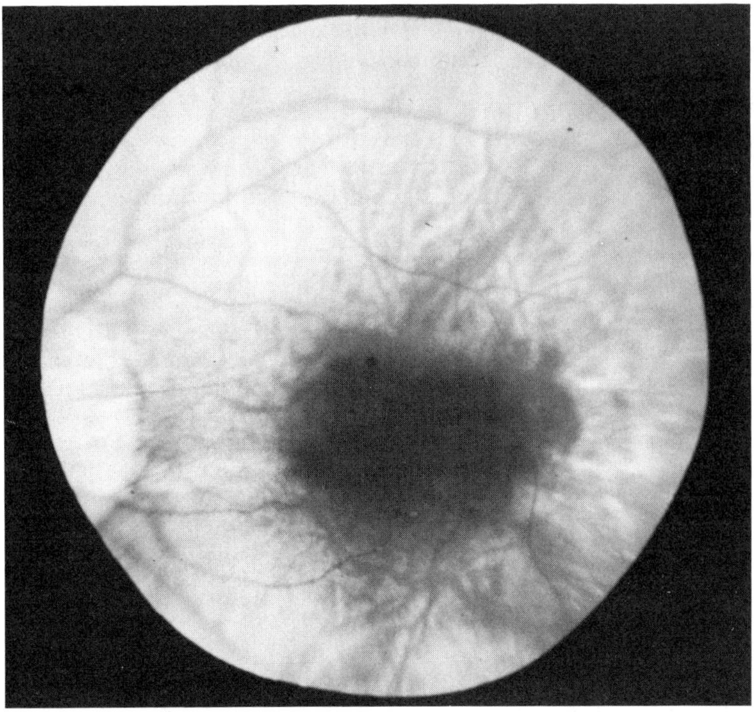

Fig. 2-8. Hemorrhage at the macula in a highly myopic eye.

"boat-shaped" hemorrhages. These most commonly arise from increased intracapillary pressure secondary to increased cranial pressure as occurs with a stroke.

Treatment

If the hemorrhage is secondary to a subretinal neovascular membrane, then treatment is as described under Degenerative Maculopathy. If the hemorrhage occurs secondary to a systemic problem, then treatment should be directed toward the systemic problem. Branch vein occlusions should have fluorescein angiography done to determine if they are ischemic or not. Ischemic vein occlusions should receive photocoagulation treatment to the ischemic area. Nonischemic vein occlusions probably do not need treatment. Recently some investigators have proposed photocoagulation treatment if cystoid macular edema occurs and persists with the vein occlusion for over 6 months.

VITREOUS HEMORRHAGE

When a patient presents in the emergency room with a vitreous hemorrhage, the first thing one must determine is whether or not the retina is attached. If there is no evidence of retinal detachment, no significantly elevated intraocular pressure, and no evidence of rubeosis iridis on the surface of the iris or in the angle, then observation is the treatment of choice. One would ask the patient to limit his activities slightly and keep his head elevated to allow the blood to settle inferiorly. Should the retina be detached including the macula (as determined by ultrasound), then one may have to do surgery to remove the blood from the vitreous and reattach the retina. Before doing any of this, one must carefully decide why the retina had detached. One additional note of caution is always to obtain a visual acuity. Any eye that has a vision of NLP (no light perception) is an eye that should not have surgery regardless of how dense the vitreous hemorrhage is. The most common causes of vitreous hemorrhage are:

1. Diabetic retinopathy
2. Posterior vitreous detachment with retinal tear
3. Posterior vitreous detachment without a retinal tear
4. Branch retinal vein occlusion
5. Trauma
6. Other causes of neovascularization of the retina
7. Macular degeneration
8. Intraocular surgery
9. Intraocular tumors

The most common cause of a vitreous hemorrhage is diabetic retinopathy. After one takes a medical history and a visual acuity, one must thoroughly inspect the iris for rubeosis. Whether or not rubeosis is found around the pupil, gonioscopy should be done on all diabetic patients. It is surprising how often rubeosis may not be found around the pupil but may be present in the angle. Obviously the rubeosis which causes us the greatest amount of trouble is that which is in the angle, since this may zipper the angle closed and cause neovascular glaucoma.

Signs and Symptoms

There is a sudden loss or deterioration of vision in the affected eye. The anterior segment may have slight cell and flare and should be carefully inspected to be sure that rubeosis iridis is not present. The normal red reflex of the fundus is diminished or absent. The fundus reflex is black rather than red. Details of the retina cannot be seen due to the cloudy media.

Treatment

Regardless of the cause of a vitreous hemorrhage, untrasound is invaluable to observe the retina. If the retina detaches, vitreous surgery becomes necessary to save the vision. The blood must be removed and surgery performed to reattach the retina. The prognosis in the case of diabetics with a vitreous hemorrhage and a traction retinal detachment is quite poor. After attempting surgical repair, approximately one in three patients sees better after surgery, one in three patients sees the same as before surgery, and unfortunately one in three patients sees worse after surgery. This is obviously a serious condition in which the results are less than impressive. For those reasons patients with extramacular traction detachment who do not have rubeosis iridis are simply followed. The risk of an extramacular traction detachment going on to involve the macula is less than 12% in the first year.

ACUTE GLAUCOMA

See Chapter 3.

TRAUMA

See Chapters 5, 6, and 9.

HYSTERIA

One must always keep in mind the possibility that a patient who comes in with a significant loss of vision and does not have an afferent pupillary defect may, in fact, be hysterical or malingering. Multiple maneuvers can be used to unveil the hysterical patient. These include "magic drops," which are instilled and followed by the suggestion that the vision will clear. During these times it is not uncommon for the patient to revert to normal or near normal vision for a brief period of time. This virtually guarantees the diagnosis. Good "magic drops" are topical anesthetics which sting slightly. Other maneuvers which may be helpful are red/green glasses on the patient with him trying to read red/green letters. The patient is not aware that he is reading certain letters with one eye and other letters with the other eye. In any event hysteria is not an emergency situation but can be time consuming.

POISONING

A wide collection of organic substances, some of which are used in industry, may cause considerable visual damage, many of them causing rapid deterioration of vision. These substances include the alcohols, especially methyl alcohol, halogens, and certain aromatic amino and nitrocompounds. Their action is on the ganglion cells of the retina or on the optic nerve fibers, causing either contraction of the peripheral field or central visual field defects, or a combination of both. There is evidence that in some cases a vascular disturbance is the initial cause. In others, the damage is neurogenic. Pathologically, the action of poisons is not well understood at present.

Ophthalmoscopic examination reveals edema of the retina and the optic disc. Occasionally, scattered hemorrhages may be seen in the retina. As the primary goal of this book is to describe ophthalmologic emergencies, we will discuss only those poisons which cause acute visual disturbances.

Methyl Alcohol (Wood Spirit, CH_3OH)

Methyl alcohol taken orally is the most common route of poisoning. Drinking only a few milliliters of methyl alcohol may produce blindness. In industrial plants poisoning may occur also by inhalation of methyl alcohol fumes. Blindness caused by cutaneous absorption is rare, but such cases have been reported.

Signs and Symptoms

The general symptoms of methyl alcohol acute poisoning are nausea, vomiting, abdominal pain, headache, and dizziness. Delirium, convulsions, and stupor may occur in severe cases. Blindness may be sudden, complete, and permanent shortly after poisoning. In certain cases, blindness is noticed on the second or third day after the ingestion of methyl alcohol. Ophthalmoscopic examination may reveal swelling of the optic disc, retinal edema, and dilatation of veins.

Treatment

Repeated gastric lavage during the first few days removes the methyl alcohol from the body. This is necessary because there is evidence that the methyl alcohol in the system continuously returns to the stomach.

Large amounts of ethyl alcohol given every few hours will protect the body against the toxic effects of methanol. This is due to preferential oxidation of ethyl alcohol by alcohol oxidase. The enzyme system is saturated with ethyl alcohol while the methyl alcohol is excreted. Ethyl alcohol treatment should be continued for a few days.

Prognosis

In less severe cases, marked improvement may occur 4-6 weeks after poisoning. Reduced visual acuity and paracentral or cecocentral scotoma are the usual final results.

Halogenated Hydrocarbons

Idoform (CHI_3) may cause loss of central vision with peripheral defect. Ophthalmoscopic changes are absent in most cases. The vision may return after discontinuance of the drug. The time of recovery varies from a few days to several months.

Methyl chloride (CH_3Cl) may cause retrobulbar neuritis, diplopia, and accommodation disturbances. Methyl bromide (CH_3Br) also causes acute visual loss. Both agents enter the human body by inhalation. Carbon tetrachloride (CCl_4) and trichlorethylene ($CHCl{:}CCl_2$) rarely cause, if at all, sudden deterioration or loss of vision.

Treatment

The treatment is mainly preventive. No effective antidote is known for poisoning by halogenated hydrocarbons.

Drugs

Chloramphenicol ($C_{11}H_{12}Cl_2N_2O_5$) is known to cause complete loss of vision after long-term administration in high doses. Most commonly, the loss of vision is due to optic neuritis or retrobulbar neuritis. Immediate discontinuation of the drug is imperative. The prognosis concerning vision is unpredictable.

Sulphanilamide ($C_6H_4(NH_2)SO_2NH_2$) occasionally may cause transient blindness. As only a few cases have been reported, not much is known about this kind of poisoning.

Quinine ($C_{20}H_{24}N_2O_2 + 3H_2O$) and quinidine ($C_{20}H_{24}N_2O_2$). Quinine is still used as an antimalarial and antipyretic drug. Its use is widely spread also for criminal abortion. Quinidine is used mainly in cardiology. Toxic effects are reported mainly from the use of quinine. The pathogenesis of quinine poisoning is not completely understood.

General symptoms include confusion of speech, tinnitus, deafness, loss of consciousness, delirium, and coma. Ocular symptom is sudden loss or severe deterioration of vision. Visual disturbances may occur after a single dose of the drug or after its prolonged administration. Visual disturbances are always bilateral, acute in nature, and of sudden onset. Vision may deteriorate rapidly and complete blindness is not unusual. The pupils are widely dilated. Fundus examination reveals contracted arteries and edematous retina. Occasionally, the picture of complete occlusion of the central retinal artery can be seen, with a cherry red spot at the macula. Quinine poisoning may be confused with hysteria; in such cases, the appearance of the fundus is the deciding factor as to whether it is quinine poisoning or hysteria.

The treatment is directed to produce vasodilatation. Retrobulbar injection of acetylcholine (200 mg), intravenous papaverine (50 mg/3-4 hr), and amyl nitrate (repeated inhalations), and priscoline 25 mg t. i. d. , are among the most commonly used vasodilators. Treatment should be started immediately after making the diagnosis. Administration of vasodilators should be continued at least for several days. If the poisoning is not severe, vision may return in a few hours. In severe cases blindness may persist for several weeks. Permanent blindness has not been reported. Peripheral visual field contraction of varying degrees is the usual end result. Central vision is the least affected. Optic atrophy is common after quinine poisoning.

Filix Mas is an anthelmintic drug, rarely used in modern medicine. The toxic dose varies from individual to individual. The drug-induced symptoms (loss of vision) may appear on the first to the twelfth day after administration of the drug. The condition may be unilateral. Loss of vision could be temporary or permanent. Ophthalmoscopy reveals constriction of retinal arteries and edema of the retina in most cases. Treatment consists of various vasodilators, as described for quinine poisoning. The prognosis of filix mas poisoning is worse than that of quinine poisoning. The end result is often constricted visual fields and optic atrophy.

Ergot taken in massive doses as an abortifacient may cause temporary amblyopia. Ergot derivatives used in obstetrics occasionally also can cause temporary deterioration of vision. General symptoms include numbness in the limbs, often followed by gangrene or convulsions. Ophthalmologic symptoms are reduced vision and peripheral contraction of the visual fields. Fundus examination reveals severe vasoconstriction and edema of the retina. The treatment is directed to produce vasodilatation. The amblyopia is transient and optic atrophy does not occur.

Salicylates and aspirin in large doses may cause temporary amblyopia. It is not clear whether the loss of vision originates in the central nervous system or if it is due to a toxic effect on the ganglion cells. General symptoms include tinnitus and deafness. Ophthalmologic symptoms, other than deteriorated vision, may include nystagmus, dilated pupils, and marked constriction of visual fields. Fundus examination often reveals constricted vessels of the retina. Treatment should concentrate on prevention of salicylate poisoning. Gastric lavage during the first few hours after salicylate or aspirin ingestion may reduce further absorption of the drug. Recovery is usually rapid. Permanent damage of vision is unusual.

BIBLIOGRAPHY

Arruga, J. et al.: Ophthalmologic findings in 70 patients with retinal embolism. Ophthalmology 89(12):1336, 1982.

Ballantyne, A. J. and Michaelson, I. C.: The Fundus of the Eye. Williams and Wilkins, Baltimore, 1970.

Barr, C. C. et al.: Acute disc swelling in juvenile diabetes mellitus. Arch Ophthal 98(12):2185, 1980.

Benson, W. E. and Spalter, H. F.: Vitreous hemorrhage. Surv Ophthal 15:297, 1971.

Blankenship, G. W. et al.: Preoperative prognostic factors in diabetic pars plana vitrectomy. Ophthalmology 89(11):1246, 1982.

Brinton, G. S. et al.: Posterior segment trauma. Amer J Ophthal 93(3):271, 1982.

Brown, G. C. et al.: Radiation retinopathy. Ophthalmology 89 (12):1494, 1982.

Charles, S. et al.: Natural history of diabetic extramacular traction retinal detachment. Arch Ophthal 99(1):66, 1981.

Clarkson, J. G.: Angioid streaks. Survey Ophthal 26(5):235, 1982.

Coltrider, N. D. et al.: Retinal emboli in mitral valve prolapse. Amer J Ophthal 90(4):534, 1980.

Cox, M. S., Schepens, C. L. and Freeman, H. M.: Retinal detachment due to ocular contusion. Arch Ophthal 76:678, 1966.

Culbertson, W. W. et al.: Acute retinal necrosis. Amer J Ophthal 96(5):683, 1983.

Dufour, D., Constantinioles, G. and Wannebroucq, C.: Action de la thrombosamine-heparine dans une thrombose arterielle retinienne. Bull Soc Ophthal Franc 68:137, 1968.

Duke-Elder, S.: System of Ophthalmology. Injuries. Vol XIV. Mosby, St. Louis, 1972.

Duke-Elder, S. and Dobree, G. H.: System of Ophthalmology. Diseases of the Retina. Vol 10. Mosby, St. Louis, 1967.

Dufour, R.: The pathogenesis of retinal detachment. Ophthalmologica 148:386, 1964.

Ellis, C. J. et al.: Medical investigation of retinal vascular occlusion. Brit Med J 2:1093, 1964.

Everett, W. G.: Bilateral retinal detachment and degenerations. Trans Amer Ophthal Soc 64:543, 1966.

Gall, J.: ACTH and cortisone administration in inducing the reabsorption of vitreous and retinal hemorrhages. Orv Hetil 101:1681, 1960.

Gass, J. D. M.: Sympathetic Ophthalmia following vitrectomy. Amer J Ophthal 93(5):552, 1982.

Gass, J. D. M.: Vitiliginous chorioretinitis. Arch Ophthal 99 (10):1778, 1981.

Gass, J. D. M. et al.: Choroidal osteoma. Arch Ophthal 96(3): 428, 1978.

Gombos, G. M.: A new treatment of central retinal artery occlusion. Ann Ophthal 2:893, 1970.

Gorman, B. D. et al.: Acute retinal necrosis. Ophthalmology 89(7):809, 1982.

Hannon, J. F.: Vitreous hemorrhages associated with sickle-cell hemoglobin C disease. Amer J Ophthal 42:707, 1956.

Hardenbergh, F. E.: Occlusion of central retinal artery. Arch Ophthal 67:556, 1962.

Hayreh, S. S. et al.: Hemi-central retinal vein occlusion. Arch Ophthal 98(9):1600, 1980.

Holland, G. N. et al.: AIDS: ocular manifestations. Ophthalmology 90(8):859, 1983.

Holland, G. N. et al.: Ocular disorders and immunodeficiency. Amer J Ophthal 93(4):393, 1982.

Jackson, R. L. et al.: Retinopathy in adolescents and young adults with juvenile onset diabetes mellitus in childhood. Ophthalmology 89(1):7, 1982.

Jampol, L. M. et al.: Peripheral proliferative retinopathies. Survey Ophthal 25(1):1, 1980.

Jalkh, A. E. et al.: Choroidal neovascularization in fellow eyes of patients with disciform degeneration. Arch Ophthal 101(8): 1194, 1983.

Jalkh, A. E. et al.: Management of subretinal neovascular membranes within the foveal avascular zone in senile macular degeneration. Amer J Ophthal 95(6):818, 1983.

Lanske, R. K.: Central retinal artery occlusion. Amer J Ophthal 60:716, 1965.

Lincoff, H., McLean, J.M. and Nano, H.: Cryosurgical treatment of retinal detachment. Trans Amer Acad Ophthal Otolaryng 68:412, 1964.

Macular Photocoagulation Study Group: Argon laser for presumed ocular histoplasmosis syndrome. Arch Ophthal 101(9): 1347, 1983.

Macular Photocoagulation Study Group: Argon laser for idiopathic neovascular membranes. Arch Ophthal 101(9):1358, 1983.

Macular Photocoagulation Study Group: Argon laser photocoagulation for senile macular degeneration. Arch Ophthal 100(6):912, 1982.

Magaral, L.E. et al.: Efficacy of panretinal photocoagulation in preventing neovascular glaucoma following ischemic central retinal vein occlusion. Ophthalmology 89(7):780, 1982.

McPherson, A. et al.: Management of fellow eyes in patients with rhegmatogenous retinal detachment. Ophthalmology 88(9): 922, 1981.

Meyer-Schwickerath, G.: Indications and limitations of light coagulations of the retina. Trans Amer Acad Ophthal Otolaryng 63:725, 1959.

Newsome, D.A. et al.: Afferent pupillary defect in macular degeneration. Amer J Ophthal 92(3):396, 1981.

Paton, B., Rubinstein, K. and Smith, V.R.: Arterial insufficiency in retinal venous occlusion. Trans Ophthal Soc U.K. 84:559, 1964.

Rice, T.A. et al.: Vitrectomy for diabetic retinopathy. Amer J Ophthal 90(3):297, 1980.

Rubinstein, K.: Arterial insufficiency in retinal venous occlusion. Trans Ophthal Soc U.K. 85:564, 1964.

Schepens, C.L., Okamura, I.D. and Brockhurst, R.J.: The scleral buckling procedures. Arch Ophthal 58:797, 1957.

Schlaegel, T.F.: Perspectives in uveitis. Annals Ophthal 13(7): 799, 1981.

Shields, J. A. et al.: Management of choroidal melanomas. Amer J Ophthal 90(2):266, 1980.

Sloas, H. A. et al.: Update of ocular reticulum cell sarcoma. Arch Ophthal 99(6):1048, 1981.

Snyder, D. A. et al.: Vogt-Koyanazi-Harada syndrome. Amer J Ophthal 90(1):69, 1980.

Tabbara, K. F. et al.: Treatment of ocular toxoplasmosis with clindamycin and sulfadiazine. Ophthalmology 87(2):129, 1980.

Watzke, R. C. et al.: Long-term course of presumed ocular histoplasmosis syndrome. Amer J Ophthal 91(6):750, 1981.

Welch, R. B. and Goldberg, M. F.: Sickle-cell hemoglobin and its relation to fundus abnormality. Arch Ophthal 75:353, 1966.

Wise, G. N., Dollery, C. T. and Henkind, P.: The Retinal Circulation. Harper and Row, New York, 1971.

Wiznia, R. A.: Natural history of senile disciform macular dystrophy. Ophthalmology 86(9):1620, 1979.

Chapter 3

EMERGENCIES DUE TO INFECTIONS OR INFLAMMATIONS

Ophthalmic emergencies due to infection or inflammation, which the physician may encounter in the emergency room or in his office, can be divided into the following:

Facial	Temporal arteritis
	Herpes zoster
Lacrimal	Dacryoadenitis
	Dacryocystitis
Orbital	Orbital cellulitis
	Cavernous sinus thrombosis
Eyelids	Herpes simplex
	Stye
	Chalazion
	Allergy
	Pediculosis
Conjunctiva	Mechanical
	Infective
	Allergy
Cornea	Mechanical
	Infective
	Allergy
Sclera	Episcleritis
	Scleritis
Uvea	Anterior
Lens	Phacoanaphylactic
Vitreous	Endophthalmitis

Retina	Central retinal artery occlusion Central retinal vein thrombosis
Optic nerve	Optic neuritis Papilledema

FACIAL

TEMPORAL ARTERITIS

Temporal arteritis usually occurs in women over age 60 having a history of severe headaches, fever, wasting, and depression.

Signs and Symptoms

Temporal arteries are tortuous, thickened, tender, and often without pulsation. Sudden loss of vision occurs in 25%. The loss of vision is due to central retinal artery occlusion which is unilateral at first, but which may become bilateral if prompt treatment is not instituted. The fundus is pale with a central cherry red spot. Arteries are narrowed. Occasionally, no retinal abnormality is seen or changes are confined to a few hemorrhages near the disc. ESR is elevated. Biopsy of the temporal artery confirms giant cell arteritis.

Differential Diagnosis

Temporal arteritis should be distinguished from retrobulbar neuritis. In the latter loss of vision is not so acute, the scotoma is usually confined to the central area; the arteries in the fundus and temple area appear normal. Temporal arteritis occurs rarely in young people, with the exception of giant cell arteritis in young Japanese women.

Treatment

Systemic steroids (80 mg/day) should be given. Emergency measures for artery occlusion (see Chapter 10) are indicated if patient presents within 24 hours of onset.

HERPES ZOSTER (Fig. 3-1)

A recent history of exposure to chickenpox may be obtained.

Signs and Symptoms

Rapid onset of fever with pain, often severe, over the area of

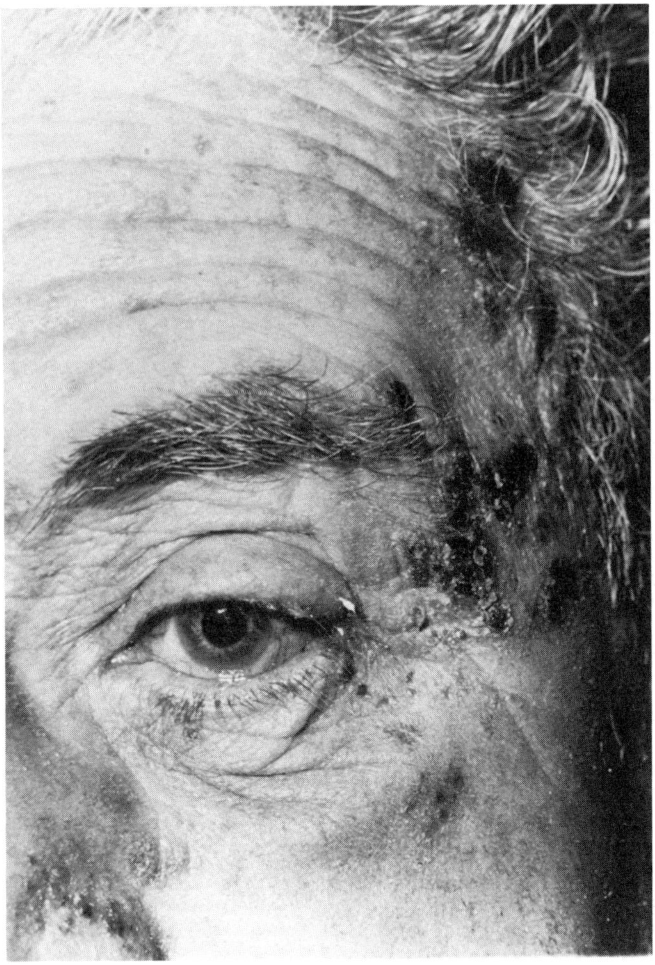

Fig. 3-1. Herpes zoster.

distribution of the first division of the fifth nerve – forehead, upper eyelid and side of the nose. These symptoms are followed in 3-4 days by a vesicular eruption in the same area. Clear fluid in the vesicles changes to yellow. The vesicles rupture leaving scars in 3 weeks. Tenderness is present over the affected area. Vesicles may occur on the conjunctiva and cornea with accompanying uveitis.

Differential Diagnosis

Herpes zoster should be distinguished from herpes simplex, which has less pain and does not show characteristic skin distribution.

Treatment

Treatment of herpes zoster is symptomatic Vitamin B_{12}(IM) and steroids may reduce the incidence of postherpetic neuralgia. Skin should be treated with bland lotions such as calamine; pain, with analgesics; and the cornea, with topical antibiotic and cycloplegics.

LACRIMAL

DACRYOADENITIS

Acute dacryoadenitis may occur in the absence of other obvious infection but it is most often seen in association with mumps, glandular fever, or gonorrhea, in which cases it is usually bilateral.

Signs and Symptoms

Dacryoadenitis presents with a feeling of fullness or pain in the upper and outer part of the upper eyelid. This is followed by edema of the outer one-third of the upper eyelid producing a characteristic S-shaped curve of the lid margin. The preauricular node may be tender and palpable. When the palpebral part of the gland is involved, palpation of the lid demonstrates a tense nut-shaped swelling separate from the orbital and lid margins. When the body of the gland is affected, an almond-shaped swelling may be felt extending under the outer orbital rim. The eye may be pushed down and inward with some proptosis often present.

Differential Diagnosis

Dacryoadenitis should be distinguished from lid abscesses and orbital cellulitis by the presence of the palpable gland.

Treatment

Treatment consists of warm compresses and analgesics. The condition usually subsides in a few days. Antibiotics may be given in the presence of known bacterial infections.

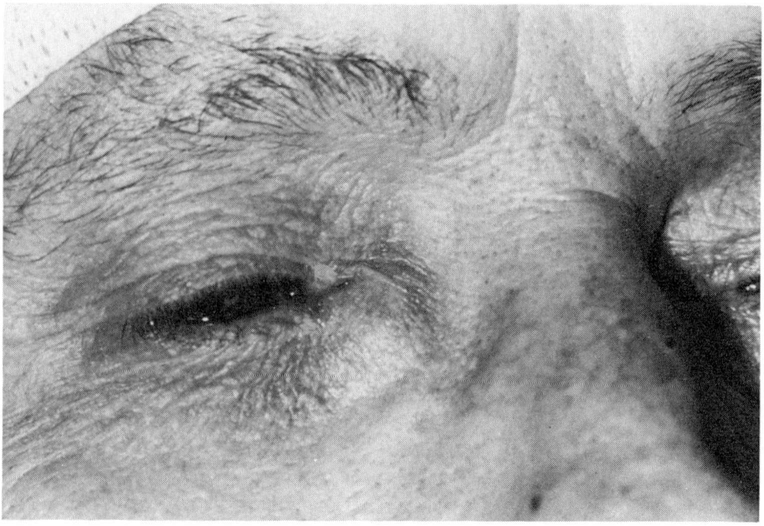

Fig. 3-2. Dacryocystitis.

DACRYOCYSTITIS (Fig. 3-2)

Infection follows blockage of tear flow from punctae, through canaliculi, sac, and nasolacrimal duct into the nose. The most common site of blockage is at the point of entry into the nose in infants and at the sac-lacrimal duct junction in adults. Both result in stagnation of the tears with consequent chronic infection in the sac accompanied by excessive tearing. Acute dacryocystitis occurs when the infection assumes a more virulent form. Tearing of the eye is usually present for some considerable time.

Signs and Symptoms

Discharge is present in the inner corner of the eye. A painful mass presents medial to the inner canthus and below the medial canthal tendon. Tender, red, sometimes fluctuant swelling may regurgitate pus from the punctae on pressure. A discharging fistula may be present on the skin surface.

Differential Diagnosis

Dacryocystitis should be distinguished from insect bite or local infection which lack tearing and discharge from eye. It also should be distinguished from lacrimal sac tumor which has less inflammation but may have blood staining of regurgitated material, and from dermoid or sebaceous cysts by lack of tearing.

Treatment

Treatment consists of hot compresses, analgesics, and systemic antibiotics adjusted for culture and sensitivity results. Dacryocystorrhinostomy is recommended after infection is controlled.

ORBITAL

ORBITAL CELLULITIS

Orbital infection is usually secondary to a nearby source, such as sinusitis or infection around the nose in the area draining into the orbital veins. Less commonly, the source may be located in the body at a distance or introduced into the orbit by a penetrating injury. A history of sinusitis or other infection is present.

Signs and Symptoms

Pain on movement of the eyes and loss of vision can occur in the later stages. Redness or swelling of one or both eyelids on one side, edema (chemosis) of the conjunctiva, and limitation of eye movement will be present. Occasionally there is double vision and displacement of the eye.

Differential Diagnosis

Rhabdomyosarcoma may occur in children. Less inflammation will be present and the eye will be increasingly displaced by the tumor. Orbital cellulitis also should be distinguished from pseudotumor which gives proptosis without pain and from unilateral exophthalmos with signs of an overactive thyroid.

Treatment

Treatment consists of systemic antibiotics in large doses.

CAVERNOUS SINUS THROMBOSIS

Cavernous sinus thrombosis occurs from infection in the venous drainage area of the sinuses, face, and nose or from orbital cellulitis, most often due to streptococcus. History includes headache, malaise, and drowsiness.

Signs and Symptoms

Fever and sometimes nausea and vomiting are present. Leucocytosis is present. These are signs of orbital cellulitis and involvement of cranial nerves II, III, IV, V, and VI.

Treatment

Treatment consists of systemic antibiotics in large doses.

EYELIDS

HERPES SIMPLEX

Herpes simplex is often associated with a febrile infection, especially inflammation of the respiratory tract. Similar lesions occur around the nares and lips. There is a history of fever and infection.

Signs and Symptoms

There is a burning sensation on one or both eyelids. Signs of herpes simplex include a pinhead-sized crop of vesicles on a swollen, slightly erythematous base filled with clear, yellowish fluid which changes to yellow-brown crusts falling off in about 7 days and leaving no scars. Herpes simplex may be associated with conjunctivitis, keratitis, and uveitis.

Differential Diagnosis

The condition should be distinguished from herpes zoster, which is more painful and has a characteristic distribution of the ophthalmic division of the trigeminal nerve.

Treatment

Treatment consists of idoxuridine (antiviral) ointment applied to lesions every 4 hours.

BLEPHARITIS

Blepharitis is an infection of the lid margins caused by invasion of the marginal glands and lash follicles by bacteria, usually streptococci. Most commonly it is a mild, chronic disease of children but occasionally it is more severe and acute in the elderly and debilitated, presenting with marginal ulcers and loss of eyelashes.

Signs and Symptoms

The patient presents with discomfort, tearing, and light sensitivity.

Treatment

Removal of the crusts is essential and is best accomplished by scrubbing the lid margins with a cotton-tipped applicator (Q-tip) which has been moistened in a bowl of warm water to which a few drops of baby shampoo have been added. This should be followed by application of an antibiotic ointment to the lid margin and repeated twice daily for several weeks.

STYE

A stye is a circumscribed acute inflammation of the lid margin due to invasion of the gland of Zeiss by staphylococci. Recurrent styes are often associated with elevated blood sugar levels.

Signs and Symptoms

There is localized pain at the lid margin. Tenderness is followed by redness and edema. The infection may point at the lid margin.

Differential Diagnosis

Stye should be differentiated from chancre with indurated margin.

Treatment

Treatment consists of hot soaks and application of antibiotic ointment to the outside and inside of lid. If the stye is centered around an eyelash, the lash should be removed. If formed, an abscess should be drained with an incision along the lid margin, not across it. Systemic antibiotics may be required if there is no response to local treatment.

CHALAZION (Fig. 3-3)

A chalazion is a distended meibomian gland in the tarsus due to blockage of its duct surrounded by inflammation. It may become secondarily infected, in which case the condition should first be treated as a stye (see above).

Signs and Symptoms

There is smooth swelling unattached to skin, adherent to the tarsus. It is well defined, like a small pea. Eversion of the eyelid may show a pale area on tarsal surface.

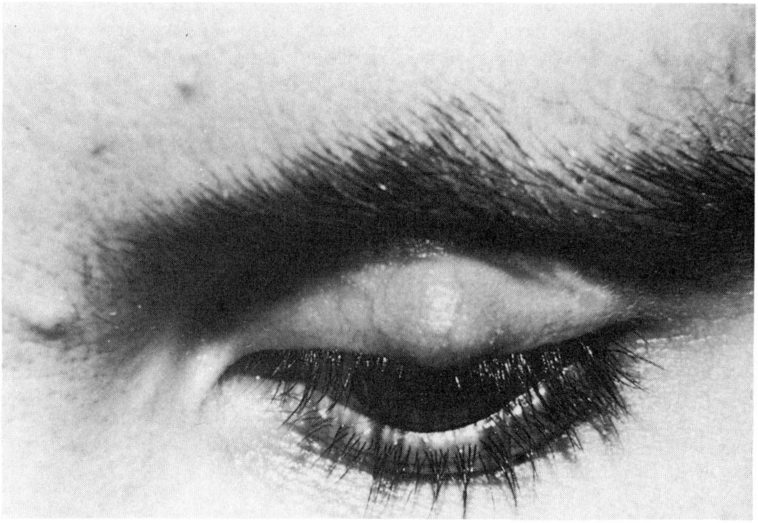

Fig. 3-3. Chalazion.

Differential Diagnosis

Chalazion should be distinguished from a stye, which is red and painful.

Treatment

Treatment consists of hot soaks followed by firm massage in the direction of the lid margin. Deposteroid should be injected into the gland. Eversion of the lid and incision and curettage through the conjunctival surface may be required.

ALLERGY

Allergy may occur due to direct contact or as a result of systemic reaction.

Signs and Symptoms

In contact dermatitis the most prominent symptom is itching. The reaction is at first erythematous but may progress to papular and pustular. Later the skin assumes a dry, shiny appearance and parchment-like surface.

Differential Diagnosis

Allergy should be distinguished from erysipelas which shows signs of inflammation, such as heat, swelling, and pain.

Treatment

The offending antigen, e. g. , drug or cosmetic, should be removed. A topical steroid should be applied twice daily to the lids (Aristocort 0. 1% cream or Valisone 0. 1% cream).

CONJUNCTIVA

BACTERIAL CONJUNCTIVITIS (Fig. 3-4)

The most common organisms encountered are *Staphylococcus pyogenes*, *Streptococcus viridans*, *Diplococcus pneumoniae*, *Corynebacterium diptheriae*, *Neisseria gonorrhoeae*, *Hemophilus influenza*, *Moraxella lacunata*, *Pseudomonas aeruginosa*, and *Proteus vulgaris*.

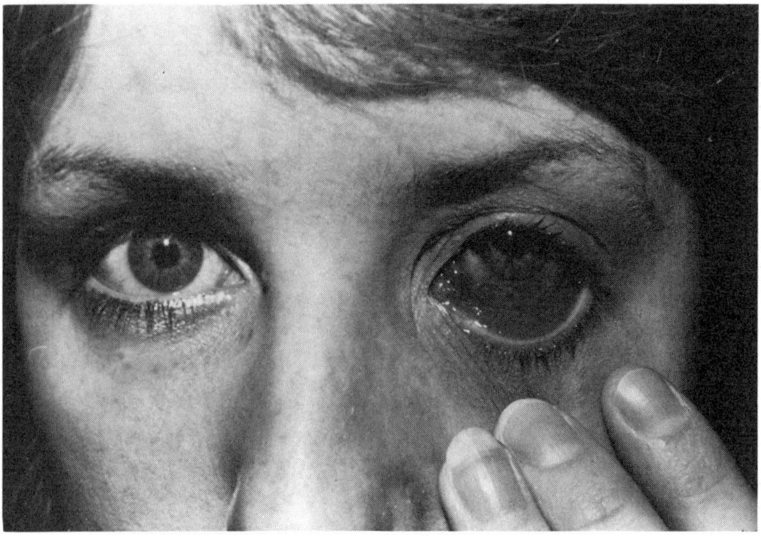

Fig. 3-4. Acute bacterial conjunctivitis.

Signs and Symptoms

The rubbing together of the inflamed palpebral and bulbar conjunctival surfaces produces a characteristic sandy or gritty sensation in the affected eye. The eye tears at first and this is followed by a mucopurulent or frankly purulent discharge. Specific questioning about the presence of a discharge upon first opening the eyes after sleep often confirms the diagnosis in mild cases. Photophobia may be present. The conjunctiva is injected. A bright red velvety appearance may develop. The inflammation usually commences in the lower fornix and spreads to the palpebral and bulbar conjunctiva. The eyelids may be swollen.

Differential Diagnosis

Subconjunctival hemorrhage produces a solid red patch on the white of the eye and is painless.

Treatment

Culture from the lower fornix is desirable before the commencement of treatment. Gram and Giemsa staining of the secretion may aid in diagnosis.

Gram-Positive	Gram-Negative
Streptococcus viridans	Neisseria gonococci
Streptococcus pneumoniae	Hemophilus influenzae
Cornynebacterium diptheriae	Proteus vulgaris
	Escherichia coli
	Moraxella lacunata

A wide spectrum of antibiotics (neomycin, gentamycin or tobramycin) should be used topically four or more times a day. In mild infections sulphacetamide or sulphasoxazole may be substituted.

OPHTHALMIA NEONATORUM

Often severe, this is a conjunctivitis occurring in the first 2 weeks after birth. Formerly almost exclusively caused by gonococci, now other organisms are more frequent including the TRIC virus (psittacocis-lymphogranuloma venereum group) which causes inclusion conjunctivitis. The cytoplasmic inclusions are visible on a Giemsa-stained smear. The onset of inclusion conjunctivitis is 5-10 days after birth, gonococcal infection is 1-5 days after.

Treatment

Both gonococcal and inclusion conjunctivitis respond to topical tetracycline therapy.

VIRAL CONJUNCTIVITIS

Signs and Symptoms

There is discomfort of the eyes with a burning sensation, tearing, and photophobia. Conjunctival injection with follicular reaction, often with marked chemosis are signs. Preauricular adenopathy may be present.

Differential Diagnosis

There is a watery discharge as opposed to purulent bacterial infection. Viral conjunctivitis is more often uniocular.

Treatment

Symptoms may be alleviated by decongestant drops of phenylephrine or naphazoline. Antibiotic drops should be prescribed to prevent secondary bacterial invasion.

ALLERGIC CONJUNCTIVITIS

Allergic conjunctivitis is often airborne and sometimes seasonal. It may accompany lid allergies. Allergy may develop to eye medications including those preparations used with contact lenses.

Signs and Symptoms

The eyes feel itchy. Conjunctival injection is present and occasionally dramatic chemosis. Vernal catarrh occurs in young people, principally males, and is characterized by seasonal incidence and the appearance of large flat-topped papillae (cobble-stones).

Differential Diagnosis

A history of exposure to allergen may differentiate from viral conjunctivitis. Discharge is mucoid when present.

CORNEA

BACTERIAL INFECTION

Infection of the cornea is often secondary to conjunctivitis and caused by the same organisms. Primary infection of the cornea is usually due to a direct injury which damages the epithelium. Few bacteria can penetrate intact epithelium (exception is Neisseria gonorrhea). Corneal ulceration which penetrates into the stroma will leave a permanent scar and visual acuity will be affected if the scar is in the optical axis.

Signs and Symptoms

There is pain in the affected eye which is often severe, as well as tearing and photophobia. Injection of the bulbar conjunctiva occurs. A discharge may be present. Visual acuity may be reduced. Using fluorescein, a greyish-white opacity staining green can be observed if the ulcer is active. The fluorescein dye is placed as a drop (from a bottle or paper strip) in the lower fornix. Blinking of the eye will then spread the dye over the cornea. The eye should be thoroughly flushed with irrigating solution before being examined for residual staining which indicates areas of epithelial loss. Ulceration of the cornea may be accompanied by the presence of a sterile inflammatory reaction in the anterior chamber. Settling of these cells may occur and present as a level white mass in the lower anterior chamber (hypopyon) (Fig. 3-5).

Treatment

Culture from the ulcer or lower fornix before commencing treatment is important. Cultures should be taken before any local anesthetic is instilled (most of these preparations are bactericidal). Gram-stained smears may aid diagnosis. A wide spectrum of antibiotics should be instilled every few hours until the organism and its sensitivity are determined. Systemic antibiotics are less effective than topical or subconjunctival administration. A cycloplegic eyedrop (hyoscine 1/4% or homatropine 2% 3 times a day) provides relief from painful iris spasm.

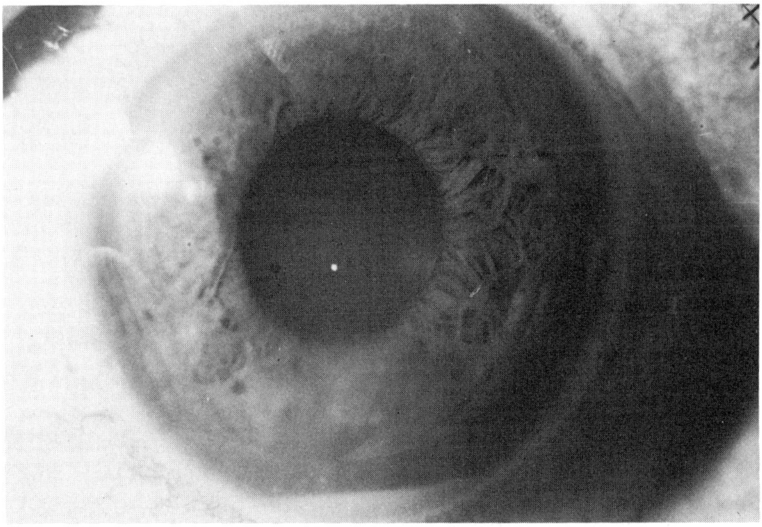

Fig. 3-5. Corneal ulcer with hypopyon.

Table 3.1

THE RED EYE

	Conjunctivitis	Uveitis	Acute Glaucoma
Vision	Normal	Reduced	Reduced
Pain	Gritty	Aching	Severe
Relief of pain with anesthetic	Yes	No	No
Discharge	Yes	No	No
Nausea	No	No	Yes
Conjunctival injection	Fornix	Limbal	Limbal
Cornea	Normal	K. P.	Steamy
Pupil size	Normal	Small	Large
Pupil reaction	Normal	Reduced	Fixed
Pressure	Normal	Normal	Elevated
Frequency	Common	Uncommon	Rare
Treatment	Topical antibiotic	Topical cycloplegic steroid	Carbonic anhydrase inhibitor miotic

VIRAL INFECTION

Among the viruses known to attack the cornea are herpes zoster, herpes simplex, and several of the adenoviruses. Herpes zoster keratitis is usually in association with an obvious skin eruption. Herpes simplex more often occurs independently of skin eruptions, though often triggered by similar factors such as a febrile episode (Fig. 3-6). The adenovirus may be accompanied by respiratory tract symptoms, and a history of contact with a "red" eye is often elicited.

Signs and Symptoms

Tearing and photophobia are prominent. Pain may be mild to severe. Circumlimbal conjunctival injection is usually present. A faint opacity or opacities may be observed on the cornea. Fluorescein staining may reveal characteristic patterns, dendritic with herpes simplex or multiple small circular dots with adenovirus.

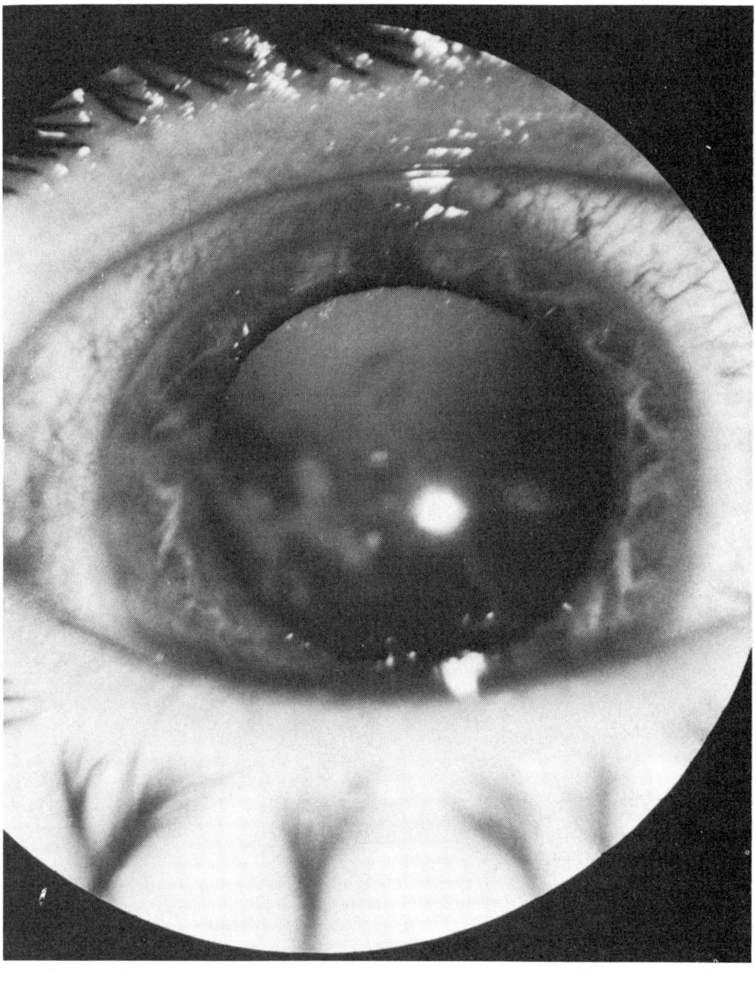

Fig. 3-6. Corneal dendritic ulcer (herpes simplex).

Treatment

Herpes zoster or adenoviral keratitis is best treated with a topical antibiotic and a cycloplegic. No specific antiviral medication is available. Herpes simplex keratitis is treated with trifluridine drops (Viroptic) or adenine arabinoside ointment (Vira-A) 4 times daily. Alternatively, idoxuridine drops or ointment (Stoxil) may be used every 2 hours.

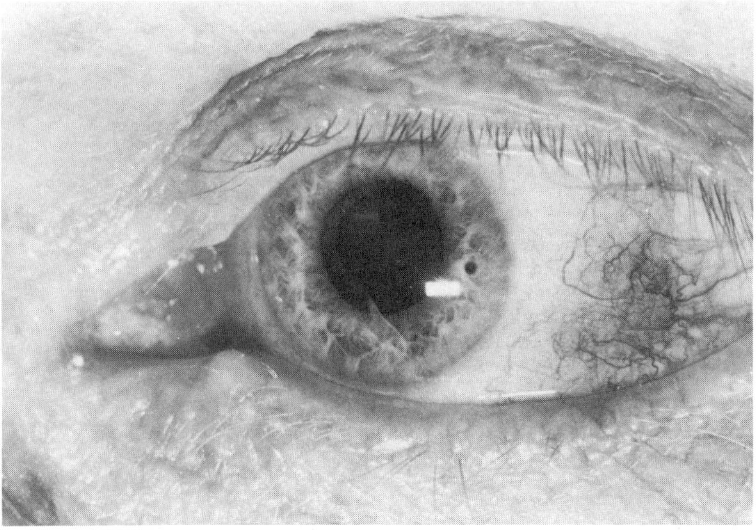

Fig. 3-7. Episcleritis.

SCLERA

EPISCLERITIS (Fig. 3-7)

The episcleral or scleral tissues may be subject to a noninfective localized lymphocytic inflammatory reaction. This is often in association with rheumatoid arthritis with similar nodules. It may be recurrent.

Signs and Symptoms

A painful nodule appears in the episcleral tissues. Vision is unaffected. The nodule is dark red or purple in color and is tender to the touch. The immediate conjunctiva is injected but the rest remains white. The deeper injection is unblanched by phenylephrine 2.5%. The conjunctiva may be moved over the deeper injection.

SCLERITIS

Signs and Symptoms

Deeper and more severe inflammation is present in the sclera. Pain may be severe, of a deep boring character. Dark red or bluish swelling in the sclera is seen, more extensively and diffusely than the nodule of episcleritis. This is accompanied by uveitis.

Treatment

Two to four hourly applications of topical steroids (prednisolone 1%, dexamethasone 0. 1%) lead to rapid relief in mild cases. Systemic administration may be needed for more severe attacks. Uveitis requires cycloplegics. Hot compresses and analgesics are used for pain.

UVEA

UVEITIS

Inflammation of the iris and ciliary body is known as anterior uveitis and inflammation of the choroid as posterior uveitis. The cause may be unknown; or the uveitis may be related to the lens, an infection in the affected eye, in the other eye (sympathetic ophthalmia), or elsewhere in the body (ranging from a tooth abscess to tuberculosis, sarcoid, or toxoplasmosis.

Signs and Symptoms

Most anterior uveitis is accompanied by pain of an aching type. Vision is reduced in the more severe cases. Injection commences as a dark red flush around the limbus before becoming more generalized. Irritation of the iris causes a small pupil (the sphincter muscle is stronger than the dilator). Cells and protein are released into the anterior chamber causing a flare when a narrow beam of light is passed through the anterior chamber. The cells may accumulate to form small round opacities visible on the back of the cornea (keratitic precipitates – Fig. 3-8). The protein released may cause the iris to adhere to the lens (posterior synechiae – Fig. 3-9). Complete adhesion around the pupil blocks the flow of aqueous. The iris is bowed forward (iris bombé), and secondary glaucoma develops. Uveitis limited to the choroid is not painful, but vision is often severely reduced since the retina and vitreous are affected and become edematous and indistinct (see Table 3. 1).

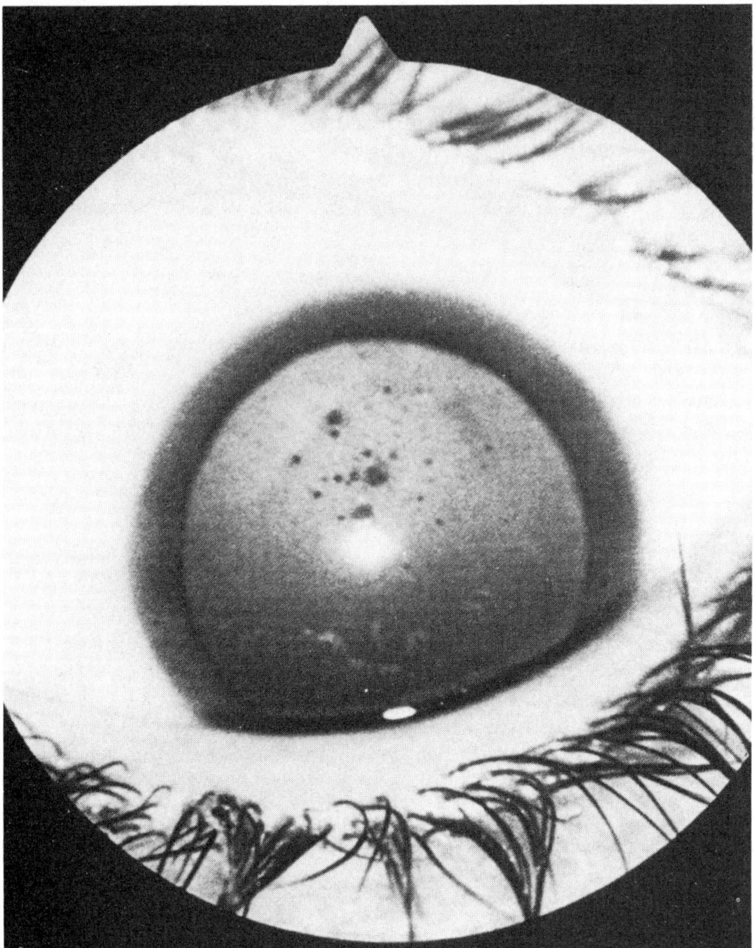

Fig. 3-8. Keratitic precipitates in uveitis.

Treatment

Topical cycloplegics (atropine 1%, hyoscine 1/4% or homatropine 2%) should be instilled 1-3 times a day. Topical steroids (prednisolone 1% or dexamethasone 0. 1%) should be given every 4 hours. Subconjunctival steroids may be necessary. Posterior uveitis requires systemic steroid therapy. A source of infection should be sought and treated if found.

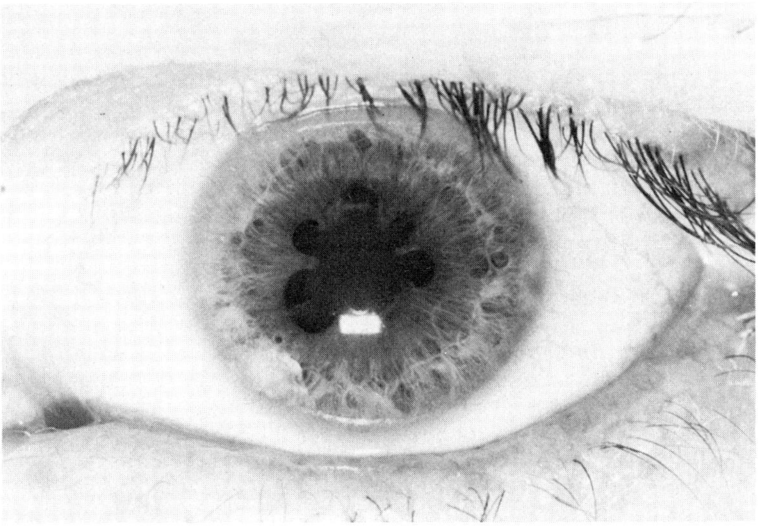

Fig. 3-9. Posterior synechiae in uveitis.

LENS

PHACOANAPHYLACTIC

Refer to section on Uveitis (above).

VITREOUS

ENDOPHTHALMITIS

Acute endophthalmitis is an inflammation within the eye usually caused by bacterial infection. The infection may reach the interior of the eye from the systemic circulation or may be introduced through a surgical or traumatic wound. The infection may be located primarily in the anterior chamber or in the vitreous or may involve both, especially in cases where the lens has been removed and aqueous and vitreous intermingle.

Signs and Symptoms

Increasing discomfort and pain occur in the affected eye. Vision deteriorates. The media of the eye become increasingly cloudy. In anterior endophthalmitis the anterior chamber fills with exudate and cells. In posterior endophthalmitis the vitreous is hazy and retinal details are obscured. The postoperative picture is one of increasing pain and visual loss instead of the normal improvement of each.

Differential Diagnosis

Endophthalmitis should be distinguished from uveitis which is uncomplicated by infection. A tap of the contents of the anterior chamber or vitreous should be done immediately if infection is seriously suspected. This will confirm the diagnosis and establish the pattern for specific treatment.

Treatment

Early treatment is essential if vision is to be saved. There is evidence that rigorous treatment including intraocular injection produces the best results. The following regimen has been suggested by Foster:

Intraocular injection of gentamicin 0.1 mg and cephaloridine 0.25 mg

Subconjunctival injection of gentamicin 40 mg and cephaloridine 100 mg

Topical gentamicin 9 mg/ml and cephaloridine or cefazolin 50 mg/ml and prednisolone 1%

Systemic cefazolin 1000 mg/6-8 hr or gentamicin 80 mg/6-8 hr

If cultures are positive, repeat intraocular injection on the second and fourth day. Subconjunctival injection every day. Topical treatment every half hour plus systemic treatment. A vitrectomy may be necessary. If cultures are negative, taper off treatment.

RETINA

See Chapter 2.

OPTIC NEURITIS

See Chapter 12.

FUNGAL INFECTIONS

Candida albicans, Actinomyces, Aspergillus, Blastomyces, Plycomycetes (mucormycosis) nocardia and Sporotrichum are causative agents occasionally found in ocular infections. Fungal ulcers of the cornea are gray, indolent and slowly progressive and often occur after injury. Hyphae of fungus can be found in scrapings and cultured on Sabouraud's Media can prove the diagnosis. Fungal infections can be treated with Amphotericin B (Fungizone) 4-10 mg/ml every 1-2 hours by eyedrops, or by subconjunctival injection 60 μg in 0.5 ml solution daily. Nystatin (Mycostatin) 100,000 units/mg ointment may be effective against Candida albicans.

BIBLIOGRAPHY

Duke-Elder, S.: System of Ophthalmology. Diseases of the Outer Eye. Vol. VIII. Mosby, St. Louis, 1972.

Duke-Elder, S.: System of Ophthalmology. The Ocular Adnexa. Vol. XIII. Mosby, St. Louis, 1972.

Henkind, P., Walsh, J. and Berger, A. (Eds.): Physicians' Desk Reference for Ophthalmology, 12th ed. Medical Economics, Oradell, NJ, 1984.

Foster, K., Abbott, R. L. and Jelender, H.: Management of infectious endophthalmitis. Ophthalmology 87:313, 1980.

Fraunfelder, F. T.: Drug-Induced Ocular Side Effects and Drug Interactions. 2nd ed. Lea and Febiger, Philadelphia, 1982.

Jones, D. B.: Chemotherapy of fungal infections. Chapter 4. In Srinivasin, B. D., Ocular Therapeutics, Masson, NY, 1980.

Chapter 4

GLAUCOMA

Glaucoma, a leading cause of preventable blindness, should be considered whenever there is a slow insidious loss of vision, whenever a red painful eye is observed or as a secondary response to other eye diseases.

The eye maintains a steady state of intraocular pressure with slight diurnal variations. This pressure is maintained by a balance between aqueous production from the ciliary body and outflow through the angle of the anterior chamber, its trabecular meshwork, Schlemm's canal and the intra- and episcleral veins. Any increase in production or obstruction to outflow can raise the intraocular pressure. This increased pressure can damage the optic nerve head either by decreasing its vascular supply or by mechanically slowing its axoplasmic flow.

The nerve fibers gradually atrophy beginning with those at the upper or lower poles of the optic disc. This results in a characteristic vertical enlargement of the cup, erosions of the rim, baring of the lamina cribosa, and displacement of the blood vessels. Many of these changes in the disc precede visual field defects. As many as 35% of the nerve fibers may be destroyed before field defects are elicited. In the more acute pressure elevations the optic nerve may develop pallor rather than the usual pattern of optic disc cupping.

CLASSIFICATION

Glaucoma can be divided into two major groups: primary glaucoma and secondary glaucoma. Primary glaucoma implies a separate disease unrelated to any other ocular or general condition. Secondary glaucoma is a consequence of another recognizable ocular or orbital disease.

Primary glaucoma can be further classified as glaucoma of the adult and glaucoma of the infant and juvenile. The adult type of glaucoma is divided into: (1) primary open-angle glaucoma (POAG), (2) acute-angle closure glaucoma (ACG), (3) combined mechanism glaucoma (CMG), and (4) congenital glaucoma (CG).

Congenital glaucoma of the infantile type is manifested during the first 3 years of life. This condition is rare. It is believed that most of these glaucomas are hereditary. Glaucoma is classified as "juvenile" when it occurs between the ages of 3 and 35. This type of glaucoma is relatively uncommon. The prevalence of glaucoma in the general population is 1.5-2% over age 35. Primary glaucoma can occur at any age; adult glaucoma occurs in individuals over 35 years of age.

The incidence of glaucoma increases with age. The majority of glaucoma cases are of the open-angle type. Acute-angle closure glaucoma comprises less than 10% of primary glaucoma cases. However, from the viewpoint of the emergency room physician, acute glaucoma is the most important type and the most likely to be encountered in ophthalmologic emergencies.

Our present classification of primary glaucoma into two main groups (POAG and ACG) originates from the gonioscopic appearance of the angle. Gonioscopy is the visualization of the angle of the anterior chamber and the trabeculum through a special contact lens. In the case of POAG, the angle is open (Fig. 4-1), while in ACG, the angle is either closed or closable. When the angle closes, the condition is associated with episodes of high intraocular pressure (Fig. 4-2).

Secondary glaucoma can be caused by many ocular conditions such as:

1. Corneal lesions with iris adherence (also called corneal adherent leucoma)
2. Uveal tract changes
    a. Anterior and/or posterior uveitis
    b. Tumor in the choroid, ciliary body, or iris

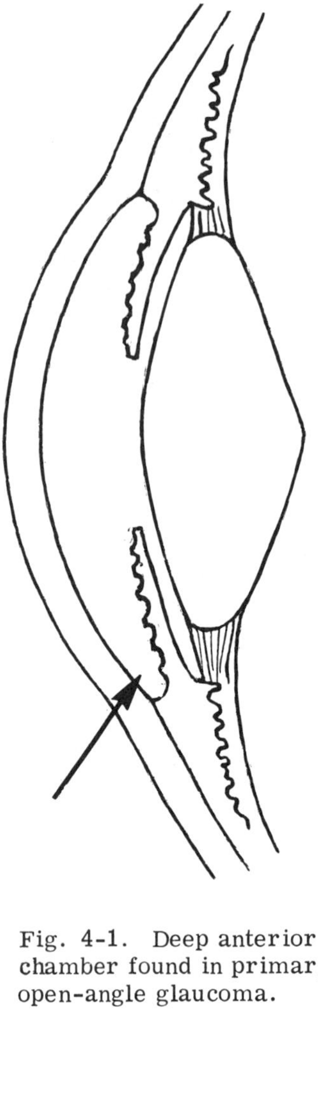

Fig. 4-1. Deep anterior chamber found in primary open-angle glaucoma.

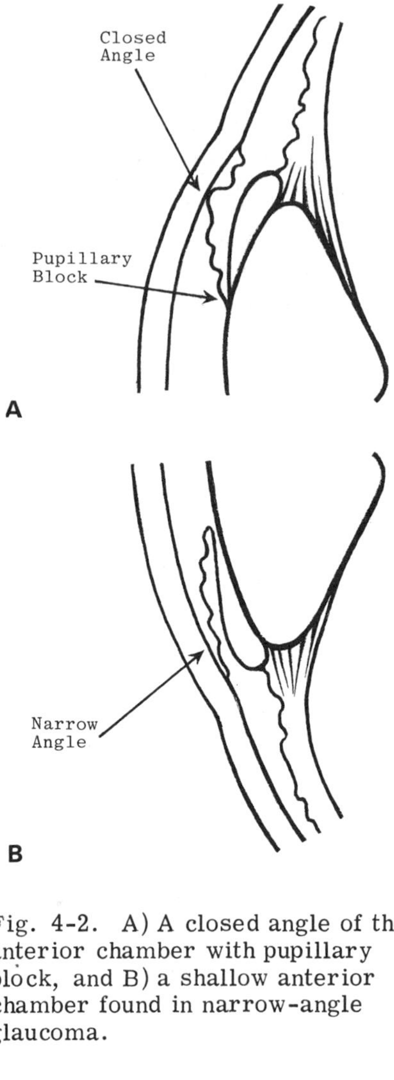

Fig. 4-2. A) A closed angle of the anterior chamber with pupillary block, and B) a shallow anterior chamber found in narrow-angle glaucoma.

c. Essential iris atrophy

3. Pathologic lens conditions
   a. Subluxation of the lens
   b. Dislocation of the lens
   c. Intumescence of the lens
   d. Phacotoxic or phacoanaphylactic reaction due to a cataractous lens

4. Trauma
   a. Hemorrhage into the anterior or posterior chamber or into the vitreous body
   b. Angle recess
   c. Hemolytic
5. Vascular conditions
   a. Central retinal vein occlusion
   b. Central retinal artery occlusion
   c. Rubeosis iridis (neovascular glaucoma)
6. Associated with use of drugs (corticosteroid induced glaucoma – topical or systemic)
7. Orbital conditions
   a. Tumor
   b. Inflammation
   c. Pulsating vascular lesions (carotic cavernous fistula)
8. Following intraocular surgery, or traumatic (perforating) injury
   a. Epithelial ingrowth
   b. Failure of reformation of the anterior chamber after intraocular surgery, and occlusion of the chamber angle by adhesions

Absolute glaucoma is present in an eye which is blind as a result of glaucoma, regardless of the type.

PHYSIOLOGIC ASPECTS OF GLAUCOMA

The intraocular pressure is determined by the rate of aqueous production by the ciliary body and by the resistance to the outflow of aqueous humor from the eye. The exact mechanism of aqueous production is not completely understood. It is most certain that the central nervous system influences aqueous production and the resistance to outflow. It is assumed that electrolytes, water, protein, and other components of the aqueous humor are produced through diffusion, ultrafiltration, and secretion, by the ciliary body and the ciliary process. From the ciliary body and the ciliary processes the aqueous humor enters into the posterior chamber. The fluid passes through the pupil into the anterior chamber. The aqueous humor leaves the anterior chamber through the trabecular meshwork and enters Schlemm's canal. Efferent channels conduct the fluid from Schlemm's canal to the venous system.

In POAG the angle is open and it is believed that the cause of the elevated intraocular pressure is the increased resistance to aqueous humor outflow. Hypersecretion is a relatively rare cause of glaucoma.

Angle-closure glaucoma occurs in an eye with a very narrow anterior chamber angle. When the pupil is dilated or the iris contracts, the root of the iris may obstruct the anterior chamber angle and this mechanical effect impairs the outflow of the aqueous humor. A pupillary block also occurs with accumulation of aqueous behind the iris, thus further compromising the angle. In combined mechanism glaucoma (CMG), there is a decreased facility of aqueous outflow associated with a tendency for angle closure.

We assume that infantile glaucoma is a result of an imperfectly developed drainage mechanism. It is believed that incomplete cleavage of the periphery of the uveal tract from the corneoscleral wall is the cause of this congenital disease. Juvenile glaucoma also results from a faulty drainage mechanism. The course is similar to that of POAG except that it is more severe in the juvenile age group.

The most important mechanism in secondary glaucoma is the increased resistance to aqueous outflow in the trabecular meshwork, the canal of Schlemm or, occasionally, the aqueous veins. Inflammatory adhesions between the iris and the lens also block the normal flow of aqueous from the posterior chamber to the anterior chamber and cause elevated intraocular pressure. Various inflammatory cells, red blood cells, protein, lens debris, and pigment can obstruct the trabecular meshwork and, in this way, cause elevated intraocular pressure. Trauma may cause injury to the trabecula (for example, atrophy, hyalinization) and be responsible for faulty aqueous outflow. The exact mechanism of elevated intraocular pressure in the case of an intraocular tumor is not well understood. The space occupied by the tumor, toxic products of the tumor, and mechanical angle closure by pushing the iris forward, are all considered to cause secondary glaucoma. In conclusion, secondary glaucoma is the state of elevated intraocular pressure associated with other ocular disease which interferes with the normal physiologic circulation of the aqueous humor.

SIGNS AND SYMPTOMS

INFANTILE GLAUCOMA

The classical triad of photophobia, blepharospasm, and tearing are the more common initial signs of infantile glaucoma. Unexplained photophobia or tearing are important signs of the disease and should not be overlooked by the physician. Corneal haze may or may not be present in the initial phase of the disease. Enlargement of the cornea or enlargement of the entire eyeball is almost always a diagnostic sign of infantile glaucoma. If the corneal diameter is larger than 12 mm, the physician should be suspicious of glaucoma. In these cases, the intraocular pressure is almost always elevated. In general, accurate tonometry cannot be performed in the emergency room. Without general anesthesia and complete rest one cannot achieve accurate measurements of the intraocular pressure of a child.

PRIMARY OPEN-ANGLE GLAUCOMA

This disease usually causes no early symptoms. Occasionally, the patient may present with dull headache when the pressure is high. When the intraocular pressure is very high and the corneal epithelium is edematous, blurred vision or a rainbow effect around lights may occur. In general, visual acuity is not affected until late in the course of the disease. Tonometry usually reveals increased intraocular pressure. External examination does not reveal any abnormality. Ophthalmoscopic examination may be normal in the early stages, but the first demonstrable changes will be found by careful study of the disc. A disparity between the cups of the two eyes may be the first hint of damage. Vertical enlargement of the cup, erosion of the rim, especially at 12 and 6 o'clock, with exposure of the blood vessels followed by baring of the lamina, bending of vessels at the disc margin and, finally, excavation of the entire disc are the sequence of glaucomatous cupping (Fig. 4-3).

ANGLE-CLOSURE GLAUCOMA

An acute attack is characterized by severe pain in or around the eye, which is usually congested. The cornea appears hazy due to edema. The anterior chamber is shallow and the pupil dilated. The vision is blurred. Gastrointestinal symptoms, such as nausea and vomiting, are often present and sometimes mask the disease. Angle-closure glaucoma does not always appear with all the above-mentioned classical signs and symptoms of the disease. Sometimes the history of pain and blurred vision only suggest the diagnosis. Occasionally, prodromal attacks may occur with minor symptoms of brow ache and slightly blurred vision. Intraocular pressure may be normal or slightly elevated between mild attacks which have been provoked by pupillary dilatation (being in darkness for a long period of time). The physician must be aware of these conditions and must know that a genuine acute attack may occur by pupillary dilatation at any time.

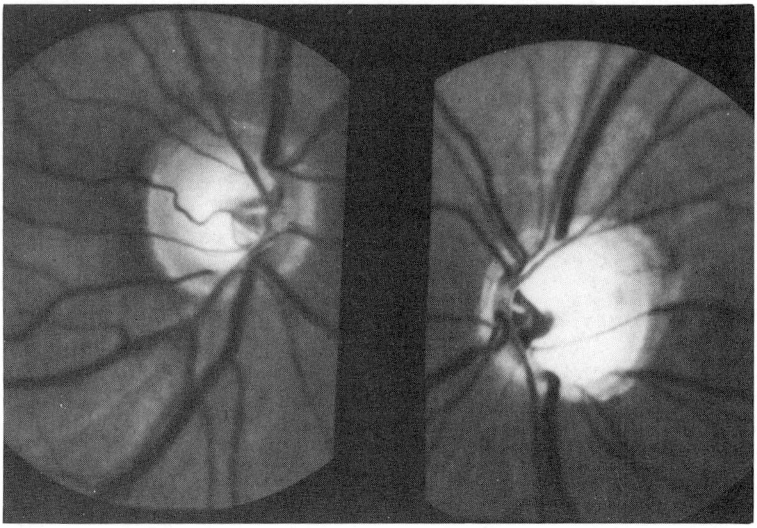

Fig. 4-3. Open-angle glaucoma with both eyes showing disparity between cups. In the right eye vessels bend into cup and are narrowed. In the left eye there is cupping to rim with vessels bending into cup at rim. There is also a nasal shift of vessels and marked pallor.

DIFFERENTIAL DIAGNOSIS OF GLAUCOMA
(Special emphasis on acute attack)

As mentioned above, primary open-angle glaucoma or infantile glaucoma is rarely presented in the emergency room. If, on occasion, such a case is encountered and the diagnosis of glaucoma is suspected, there is always enough time to refer the patient to the ophthalmologist for further evaluation. Therefore, the differential diagnosis is not discussed in this framework.

The following must be considered in the differential diagnosis of an acute attack of glaucoma: acute iritis, acute iridocyclitis, and acute conjunctivitis. In acute iritis or iridocyclitis, the pupil is constricted (not dilated), the photophobia is more pronounced, and the pain is less severe than in acute glaucoma. In acute conjunctivitis there is little or no pain, the visual acuity is unchanged, and the pupil reacts to stimulus.

Acute glaucoma can be easily overlooked when the gastrointestinal symptoms of glaucoma are very severe and mimic an acute abdominal condition. The same is true in the case of a patient with an abdominal condition which was treated with atropine or atropine-like medication and the systemic medication precipitates the acute attack of glaucoma. An eye having a narrow angle and treated for any reason with mydriatics or cycloplegics also can develop an acute attack as a result of the medication.

EMERGENCY TREATMENT

Emergency treatment is indicated only in an acute attack of angle-closure glaucoma (closed-angle glaucoma) or a severe case of secondary glaucoma. Medical therapy should be administered whenever possible. If pressure is very high, the intraocular pressure should be reduced by oral or intravenous administration of carbonic anhydrase inhibitors or hyperosmotic agents. Once the pressure is reduced below 50, the pupil will be more responsive to miotics (parasympathomimetic cholinergic agents).

1. Pilocarpine 1%-2% eyedrops are used as soon as the diagnosis is established. The drops can be instilled every 10 minutes.

2. Timolol maleate (a beta blocker) 0.5% instilled topically may reduce the production of aqueous and help lower the pressure.

3. Corticosteroid eyedrops are used to reduce inflammation.

4. Application of pressure to central cornea with a wet cotton-tipped applicator may force aqueous toward the angle and break the pupillary block.

TOPICAL TREATMENT

Miotic agents retract the iris from the corneoscleral wall and reopen the anterior chamber angle. This allows the aqueous to leave the eye through the physiologic route.

If the acute attack has been present for a few hours, the iris muscle may not respond to miotic drops and the pupil will remain dilated. Strong miotics such as isofluophate (DFP) or echothiophate (Phospholine iodide), strong anticholinesterase drugs, cause congestion of the iris stroma and the ciliary body and, therefore, should be avoided. For this reason, in an acute attack many ophthalmologists do not use pilocarpine in concentrations higher than 2%, or eserine higher than 1%.

SYSTEMIC TREATMENT

Often, the patient suffering from an acute attack of glaucoma is nauseous. Therefore, the intravenous route of medication may be necessary.

Acetazolamide (Diamox), 500 mg IV, should first be administered. This medication should be continued with a dose of 250 mg/4 hours by mouth after the nausea has subsided. Practically, there is no known contraindication to this kind of medication except proved hypersensitivity to the drug. Diamox is a carbonic anhydrase inhibitor. It reduces the production of the aqueous humor and in that way reduces also the elevated intraocular pressure. Other carbonic anhydrase inhibitors such as methazolamide (Neptazane) and dichlorphenamide (Daranide) may also be used in an acute attack.

Glycerol is one of the more commonly used hyperosmotic agents. It is administered by mouth. It is safe and it can be given even in the ophthalmologist's office. The usual amount is 1 ml/kg body weight in 50% solution. Its main advantage is its easy use. However, if the patient is nauseous or vomiting, often he will not tolerate glycerol. Glycerol is metabolized as a carbohydrate and so may cause hyperglycemia and glycosuria. If it is administered intravenously, in error, it can cause hematuria by damaging the afferent glomerular arterioles.

The combination of miotics, carbonic anhydrase inhibitor, and hyperosmotic agent is the best and most effective combined medication to treat an acute attack of glaucoma. After intensive treatment, the intraocular pressure will usually fall to normal level within 30 minutes to a few hours. The visual acuity improves gradually. Miotic drops such as pilocarpine should be continued every 4 hours. Miotics also should be instilled in the fellow eye to avoid the danger of an acute attack in that eye.

Mannitol is a hyperosmotic agent. It is administered intravenously in amounts of 1.5-2.0 g/kg body weight in 20% solution. Before the start of this treatment the physician should check the patient's heart condition to determine whether he can tolerate the required amount of medication. The total amount of mannitol is given during a 1-hour period. Prior to administration the mannitol solution should be checked for the presence of crystals. If crystals are present, warming the bottle containing the solution will eliminate the crystals in the fluid. Mannitol is not metabolized in a significant amount and, therefore, it can be used safely in the presence of diabetes.

Urea (Urevert) is another hyperosmotic agent. It also is administered by intravenous route in amounts of 1 g/kg body weight. This medication is extremely effective; however, its use is contraindicated in patients suffering from liver or kidney disorders.

FINAL TREATMENT

An acute attack of angle-closure glaucoma almost certainly will reoccur if the eye is not operated on. Therefore, after successful treatment of the first acute attack of glaucoma, the patient's eyes should be examined and evaluated by an ophthalmologist. Gonioscopy should be performed. Surgical treatment, either laser iridotomy, laser iridoplasty, or peripheral iridectomy, should be done as soon as the condition of the eye is suitable for surgery.

TREATMENT OF SECONDARY GLAUCOMA

In general, the patient appears in the emergency room with this type of glaucoma because of severe pain or the previously mentioned signs of an acute attack of glaucoma, namely, nausea, vomiting, and blurred vision. The treatment of secondary glaucoma is almost as varied as the cases. Thus, the treatment must be divided into two main groups: treatment of the underlying disease and treatment of the elevated intraocular pressure.

The emergency room physician must concentrate his efforts to relieve the acute symptoms and to reduce the patient's discomfort. To reduce intraocular pressure, carbonic anhydrase inhibitors and hyperosmotic agents are safe and helpful drugs. In certain cases, sympathomimetic eyedrops such as Neosynephrine 10% can be used to reduce aqueous humor production and, in that way, also the intraocular pressure.

Five hundred mg of Diamox are administered intravenously.

Intravenous administration of the drug provides quick action. Diamox should be continued in a dose of 250 mg 4 times/day by mouth. Mannitol, urea, or glycerol could be added. The dosage and the contraindications for treatment of an attack of secondary glaucoma are the same as those mentioned previously for acute closed-angle glaucoma. It is advisable not to administer pilocarpine drops unless the etiology of the secondary glaucoma is clear. Pilocarpine causes vasocongestion and might worsen the condition of the underlying disease responsible for the elevated intraocular pressure. The patient might benefit with local treatment of epinephrine, norepinephrine 1% eyedrops (Eppy, Glaucon) or Neosynephrine 2. 5% or 10%, cycloplegics, timolol, and corticosteroids.

FINAL TREATMENT

The type of treatment varies according to the etiology of the secondary glaucoma. The glaucoma that accompanies some inflammations of the eye, such as iritis and iridocyclitis, may benefit quickly from corticosteroids and cycloplegic eyedrops. Others, such as pupillary block, need surgical intervention (iridectomy) to provide prompt relief. Glaucomas that develop due to closure of main blood vessels of the eye can be quite resistant to treatment and sometimes the decision is difficult as to whether to be conservative or to operate on the eye. One principle must be remembered by the physician seeing and treating the patient with a secondary glaucoma: administration of different kinds of medication, except those reducing the intraocular pressure (Diamox, glycerol), should not be done until the proper diagnosis has been established.

BIBLIOGRAPHY

Becker, B. and Shaffer, R. N.: Diagnosis and Therapy of the Glaucomas, 3rd ed. Mosby, St. Louis, 1983.

Chandler, P. A. and Grant, W. M.: Glaucoma. Lea and Febiger, Philadelphia, 1979.

Newell, F. W.: Ophthalmology – Principles and Concepts, 5th ed. Mosby, St. Louis, 1982.

Quigley, H. A., Hohman, R. M., Addicks, E. M., Massof, R. W. and Green, R. W.: Morphologic changes in the lamina cribrosa correlated with neural loss in open-angle glaucoma. Am J Ophthal 95(5):673-91, 1983.

Scheie, H. G. and Albert, D. M.: Adler's Textbook of Ophthalmology. W. B. Saunders, Philadelphia, London, Toronto, 1969.

Chapter 5

TRAUMA: PART I – NONPENETRATING AND NONPERFORATING INJURIES OF THE EYEBALL

Trauma of the eyeball is relatively common despite the well-developed protective mechanism of the visual system. The bony orbital rim prevents many injuries of the eyeball itself. The eyelashes and eyelids are highly sensitive and the lids quickly close reflexively through stimuli. In this way, serious injury to the globe is prevented. The upward rotation (Bell's phenomenon) of the eye due to a sudden stimulus is an additional reflexive action which helps protect the cornea from injury.

It should be understood that in many cases the eye might have useful vision if careful attention were provided immediately after the injury. Therefore, the emergency room physician should be familiar with the treatment of a traumatized eye. An ocular injury requires immediate attention, diagnosis, and definitive treatment. Very often, proper first-aid attention can prevent future complications and further deterioration of the condition of the eye. Improper handling and poor management can destroy an injured eye and can cause permanent blindness.

Ocular injuries can be divided into two groups: nonpenetrating injuries and penetrating and perforating injuries of the eyeball. In this chapter, we shall discuss nonpenetrating and nonperforating injuries. Nonpenetrating injuries include: superficial injuries of the cornea (abrasion, foreign body); chemical and physical injuries; and contusion and concussion injury of the eyeball.

SUPERFICIAL CORNEAL INJURIES

ABRASION OF THE CORNEA

Traumatic removal of corneal epithelium is called abrasion of the cornea. This condition may be due to friction from a foreign body in the conjunctival sac or on the cornea, or it may be caused by a variety of abrasive injuries. Commonly seen are scratches from paper, brushes, finger nails, and many other household items. Flying objects may injure the corneal epithelium without adhering to the cornea. A corneal abrasion is usually not a serious condition. There is, however, a tendency for recurrence weeks or even months after the injury has healed.

Signs and Symptoms

The patient may complain of foreign body sensation and photophobia. Abrasion may cause severe pain. Lacrimation, blepharospasm, and blinking of the eyelid are common signs of corneal abrasion. The conjunctiva is usually hyperemic. Visual acuity may be normal or only slightly deteriorated.

Examination

Examination of the cornea by direct bright light may be negative. The epithelial injury or denudation of the cornea, however, is easily seen when fluorescein dye is instilled into the conjunctival sac. Occasionally, the examination of an eye so injured is difficult. In order to facilitate the examination, the pain associated with the abrasion can be relieved by instillation of local anesthetic eyedrops, such as proparacaine hydrochloride 0. 5% (Ophthaine).

Instillation of local anesthetic should not be continued since it delays the reepithelization of the cornea and masks the diagnosis of possible complications such as infection or anterior uveitis which might cause continuous pain.

Treatment

Any debris present in the conjunctival sac should be removed. Administration of a short-acting cycloplegic such as tropicamide 1% (Mydriacyl) or cyclopentolate 0. 5% (Cyclogyl) eyedrops is advisable. This will make the eye more comfortable and will reduce secondary iridocyclitis. A broad-spectrum antibiotic such as chloromycetin 1%, drops or ointment, will prevent potential bacterial infection. An eye patch is applied with gentle pressure for 1 or 2 days. Corneal abrasion heals relatively quickly, usually within 1-3 days; however, daily examination is required. If Bowman's membrane is not damaged, no sign of corneal abrasion will remain after injury.

SUPERFICIAL FOREIGN BODIES

A foreign body such as a glass, wood, or metallic particle may be propelled into the eye by moving machinery (Fig. 5-1). A foreign body also may drop into the eye, or the wind may blow it on the cornea. Multiple foreign bodies may be driven into the cornea by an explosion. The retention of a foreign body on the surface of the eye is the most common ocular injury caused by accident. Organized material causes considerable irritation. A foreign body such as grain may excite an irritative inflammatory reaction with edema and discharge. On the other hand, glass, plastic, or stone may be seen on the cornea without significant reaction.

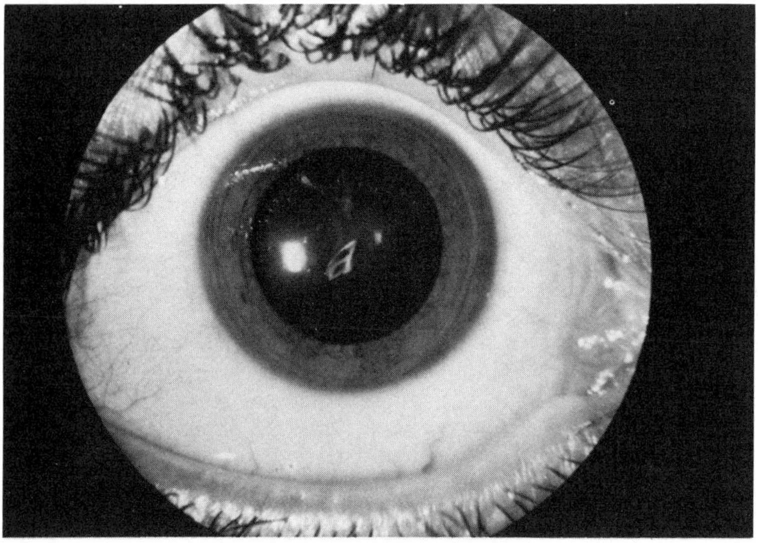

Fig. 5-1. Superficial corneal foreign body.

Signs and Symptoms

The patient suffers from pain, lacrimation, and foreign-body sensation. Repeated blinking may be observed and the visual acuity is reduced. The conjunctiva is hyperemic. If the foreign body has been in the cornea for a long period of time, photophobia may be present. Examination of the cornea, using an oblique moving bright light, may reveal the foreign body. A metallic foreign body is surrounded by a rust ring within a relatively short period of time.

Treatment

Administration of topical anesthesia is necessary for removal of a foreign body imbedded in the cornea. Proparacaine, 0. 5%-1% (Ophthaine) or tetracain (Pontocaine) eyedrops instilled 3-4 times into the conjunctival sac provide adequate anesthesia. Removal of a foreign body is best accomplished with a small, sharp instrument. A sterile hypodermic needle is satisfactory as is a special foreign body removal spud. The average superficial particle can be dislodged easily with only minimal damage to the surrounding tissue. One must remember that the cornea is thin (less than 1 mm) and, therefore, care must be taken not to perforate it. A cotton-wool applicator is an unsatisfactory instrument for this purpose. It causes extensive damage to the surrounding epithelium and is not suitable to remove rust rings around a metallic foreign body. An unremoved rust ring behaves as an unremoved foreign body and continues to irritate the eye. Therefore, both the foreign body and the rust ring must be removed. When the rust ring is deeply embedded, it might be better to patch the eye for 24 hours and remove the rust ring after it softens. This is best accomplished on the slit lamp.

After removal of the foreign body, a short-acting cycloplegic such as tropicamide 1% (Mydriacyl), or cyclopentolate 0. 5% (Cyclogyl) eyedrops will reduce the effects of secondary iritis. A broad-spectrum antibiotic ointment such as 1% chloromycetin or gentamicin should be used and an eye patch should be applied with gentle pressure for one to several days.

Daily examination of the injured eye and application of an antibiotic and a cycloplegic should be continued until the corneal wound is completely healed. Many ophthalmologists do not patch an eye after removal of a foreign body because patching encourages infection. However, the patient feels more comfortable with a pressure-patch and, therefore, patching is advisable for a few days. Many ophthalmologists use antibiotic drops only, since ointments delay wound healing. However, antibiotic ointment gives better protection against infection since it remains in the conjunctival sac for a longer period of time and, therefore, its use is recommended.

To summarize the treatment in steps:

1. Remove the foreign body (including the rust ring)
2. Administer a cycloplegic
3. Administer an antibiotic
4. Patch the eye

CHEMICAL INJURIES

Chemical burns are quite common. They can be caused by either acid or alkali. They may occur in laboratory, industrial, or household accidents. Regardless of the type of causative agent, chemical burns need immediate attention. An acid immediately precipitates the superficial tissue proteins and generally does not penetrate deeply into the eye. The damage is limited to the superficial layers of the cornea or conjunctiva and is immediate. There are no later effects such as cell disruption or tissue softening. On the other hand, alkali burns are much more serious. Alkali penetrates the cornea, the anterior chamber, and even the retina within a very short period of time. Penetrating alkali disrupts living cells and softens the tissue. Laboratory experiments show that an alkali-burned cornea contains broken-down collagen. The extent of injury of a chemical burn is related to the nature and concentration of the chemical agent. In general, the higher the alkali pH, the more serious is the injury.

SIGNS AND SYMPTOMS

In general, not only the conjunctiva and the cornea, but the eyelids and the surrounding skin also are involved in a chemical injury. The skin and the lids can be whitish (pale) and appear necrotic. Coagulation of the corneal tissue causes opacity of the cornea which, therefore, appears to be whitish and opaque (Fig. 5-2). The conjunctiva, if severely injured, is pale because it is ischemic. Blanching of the limbus signals increasing severity of the injury. Pain can be severe or none at all depending on the damage of the sensory elements of the cornea. In most cases, the vision is severely impaired.

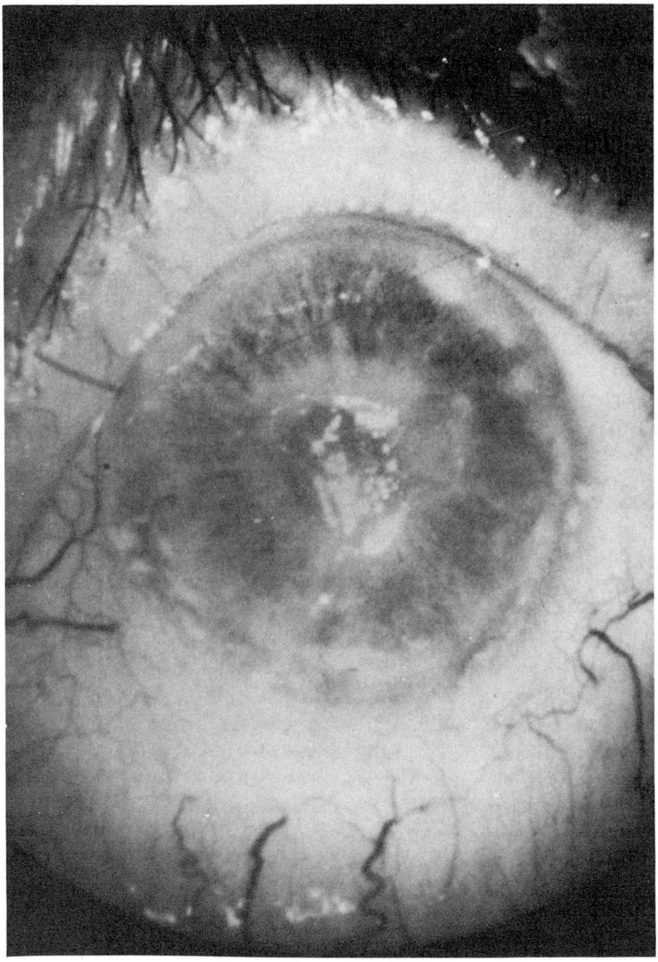

Fig. 5-2. An eye 2 months after an alkali burn. The cornea is white and vascularized.

TREATMENT

Irrigation of the eyes and the surrounding tissue is the immediate treatment for chemical burns. As more time elapses between injury and decontamination, the prognosis worsens. One should not wait for a sterile, physiologic mild acid or alkali solution, but should wash out the chemical agent with tap water immediately. The fornices of the conjunctivas must be swept with wet cotton applicators; the eyelids should be everted and washed. Solid particles or crystals should be removed either by a cotton applicator or by a pair of forceps. Most ophthalmologists do not recommend irrigation for a long period of time if acid is the chemical agent causing the injury.

In the case of an alkali burn, the initial lavage should be followed by continuous irrigation with physiologic solution. At least 1000-2000 ml of normal saline 0. 9% should be used for at least 1 hour. A convenient approach is running normal saline (0. 9%) via IV tubing into the eye. It was recently demonstrated that irrigation for long periods of time does not eliminate any more chemical agents from the ocular tissues. The best advice is to examine the pH in the conjunctival sac; if it is alkaline, continue the irrigation until the pH is restored to normal, or at least close to normal (tears have a pH of between 7. 3 and 7. 7). Urine pH sticks are useful for this purpose.

After lavage, cycloplegics, mydriatics, and antibiotics are administered into the conjunctival sac. Atropine 1% or hyoscine 0. 3%, and Neosynephrine 10% eyedrops are used to dilate the pupil and to prevent massive adhesions between the lens and the iris (posterior synechiae); they also reduce the symptoms of secondary iridocyclitis. Chloromycetin, bacitracin, or Garamycin eye ointment is applied to prevent infection. Discomfort may be reduced with occasional administration of topical anesthetics. Frequent use of topical anesthetics is not recommended since they inhibit healing. If the pain is severe, systemic analgesics should be administered, the injured eye should be patched, and the patient must be hospitalized. The use of topical corticosteroids in chemical injuries is controversial and may be used only under the direct observation of an ophthalmologist.

COMPLICATIONS AND PROGNOSIS

Chemical burn caused by acid has a relatively good prognosis. The cornea and conjunctiva may be damaged seriously but the posterior segment of the eye rarely suffers from the injury. The ultimate prognosis of vision is relatively good.

Alkali burns are serious. Extensive destruction of conjunctiva and cornea is not unusual. In an alkali-burned cornea, collagenase is produced by cells which repopulate the damaged cornea (that is, epithelium). Collagenase attacks unprotected collagen of the cornea which causes ulceration or even perforation of the cornea. For this reason, collagenase inhibitors are used in the alkali-burned cornea starting 1 week after injury. Cysteine or acetylcysteine is used by many ophthalmologists. Cysteine is administered as a 0. 2 molar solution, a few drops every 4 hours.

The outer layers of the ocular tissue as well as the inner aspect may suffer severely from the chemical agent; alkali may penetrate into the retinal tissue and destroy all the sensory elements, thus causing complete blindness. In general, chemical burns are not treated surgically in the emergency room. Tissue destruction becomes evident only a few days later. Surgery is usually not indicated during the first few weeks following an alkali burn. The only surgery of an emergency nature is therapeutic corneal graft after corneal perforation. Replacement of conjunctiva by buccal mucosa or corneal graft for optical reasons can be performed only several months after injury. Complicated cataract or secondary glaucoma is a common complication after chemical injuries. Surgery of any kind for alkali burns has a very poor prognosis.

PHYSICAL INJURIES

ULTRAVIOLET RADIATION

Ultraviolet radiation is the most common form of radiation injury. Natural sunshine, sunlamps, and welding arcs are the more common causes of this type of injury. Usually the corneal epithelium is injured. The prognosis of such an injury is good. Permanent impairment of vision from ultraviolet radiation is not common.

Signs and Symptoms

The patient presents with severe pain, photophobia, and blepharospasm usually several hours after exposure. The latent period between the time of injury and the appearance of the symptoms may be from 6 to 10 hours. The conjunctiva is chemotic and diffuse punctate fluorescein staining of the cornea is present. Visual acuity may be normal or slightly deteriorated. Diffuse corneal haze may be seen in a severe case of industrial injury. Spastic miosis may develop. The pain may be relieved by the application of topical anesthetics for a short period of time.

Treatment

Short-acting cycloplegic drops such as tropicamide 1% (Mydriacyl) or cyclopentolate 0.5% (Cyclogyl) should be administered to relieve pain due to secondary iritis. Topical antibiotic drops or ointment such as chloromycetin, bacitracin, or neomycin will prevent infection. The eye should be patched for 24 hours. If both eyes are severely injured, then bilateral patching is indicated. Analgesics also should be used to relieve the pain.

INFRARED RADIATION

Prolonged exposure to infrared radiation occasionally may produce superficial keratitis. The so-called glassblower cataract is caused by multiple exposures of infrared radiation, but this is not considered an ocular emergency.

Signs, Symptoms, and Treatment

The signs, symptoms, and treatment of infrared radiation are the same as those of ultraviolet radiation.

THERMAL BURNS

Thermal burns usually effect the eyelids. Marked edema and redness of the lids are seen. Because of the lid reflex closure, the cornea is rarely affected. Accidents arise from flying objects such as the lighted end of a cigarette. If the lid burn is so severe that lid closure is impaired, the exposed cornea must be covered with antibiotic ointment until a plastic surgery procedure can be performed to replace the destroyed tissue. A corneal burn should be treated with topical antibiotics and short-acting cycloplegics.

IONIZING RADIATION

Exposure of tissue to ionizing radiation is always followed by a latent period before any sign of reaction occur. The latent period varies and depends on the dose of radiation. Occasionally, clinical symptoms occur several weeks after injury; thus, ionizing radiation is not always an emergency. The conjunctiva and the cornea are considered to be more radiosensitive than other tissues. The lens, uvea, retina, and optic nerve also may suffer from ionizing injury.

Signs and Symptoms

The conjunctival reactions to radiation are hyperemia, circumcorneal injection, and watery discharge. Mucopurulent discharge is not an uncommon complication. Visual acuity may be normal or deteriorated.

The earliest clinical sign of radiation damage of the cornea is hypoasthesia. Radiation keratitis results in the loss of epithelium resembling superficial punctate keratitis or superficial ulcers. Occasionally, interstitial keratitis and aseptic corneal necrosis may develop. Clinical lesions of the uvea include vascular dilatation and tissue edema. Hemorrhages in the retina, papilledema, and thrombosis of the central retinal vein are very rare complications of radiation injury. Radiational cataract is always a late complication. The first clinical sign if the appearance of pepper-like opacities at the posterior pole of the lens in the plane of the capsule.

Treatment

The treatment of radiation injuries is symptomatic. A cycloplegic such as Cyclogyl 1% or homatropine 5% and an antibiotic such as chloromycetin 1% or gentamicin 1% should be administered to reduce signs of active iritis and to prevent infection. Frequent administration of artificial tears will help treat the keratitis.

CONTUSION AND CONCUSSION INJURY TO THE EYEBALL

Contusion and concussion injury can be classified as follows: contusion injury, concussion injury due to tissue conduction, and concussion injury due to air conduction. Contusion injury of the eye is damage caused by direct contact with the eyeball by any one of a large variety of blunt objects, for example, a stone striking the eye directly, or a fist. Concussion injury refers to a blow not directly striking the eye. An injury to the head is the most common cause of concussion injury of the eye by tissue conduction. The striking force hits the head and the waves of this force are conducted to the eye through tissue, namely the bone and the orbital fat. Concussion injury conducted by air occurs in the case of an explosion. The waves come from an explosion far away from the eye. The waves hit the cornea and are transmitted to the other ocular tissues, causing many kinds of injury to the eyeball.

The results of contusion and concussion injuries are variable. They may cause damage to the anterior segment of the eye as well as the posterior segment. Very often the extent of damage shortly after injury is unknown. Careful follow-up is necessary in most cases to evaluate the final damage. Some signs such as hemorrhage or dislocated lens are evident immediately after injury; however, others, such as cataract, may develop later. The emergency room examination must first exclude the possibility of rupture of the eyeball. (Signs of perforating injury are described in Chapter 6.)

Contusion or concussion injury may cause:

1. Ecchymosis, subconjunctival hemorrhage (Fig. 5-3)
2. Corneal lesions (opacities and rupture of membranes)
3. Hyphema
4. Iridodialysis, traumatic aniridia, changes in accommodation and refraction, and changes in the pupil
5. Ciliary body detachment and traumatic iridocyclitis
6. Recession of the anterior chamber angle and other conditions causing concussion glaucoma
7. Subluxation or dislocation of the lens and cataract
8. Herniation of the vitreous into the anterior chamber
9. Vitreous hemorrhage
10. Rupture of the choroid, hemorrhage of the choroid, and traumatic choroiditis
11. Retinal hemorrhage and edema
12. Retinal detachment
13. Rupture of the eyeball

These injuries may appear separately or in combination.

ECCHYMOSIS, SUBCONJUNCTIVAL HEMORRHAGE

Ecchymosis is a contusion injury of the eyelids. Hemorrhage and edema are present in the eyelids. No special treatment is required if these are the only conditions present. The hemorrhage and edema will disappear gradually within a few weeks.

Hemorrhage from conjunctival and episcleral vessels may occur without any or with only minimal laceration of the conjunctival tissue. Sometimes a large amount of blood coagulates under the conjunctiva causing a black ring around the cornea. Surgical evacuation of such a clot is very often unsuccessful. The hemorrhage will dissolve within 2 weeks. No special treatment is required for this condition. The use of antibiotic drops or ointment is advisable to prevent possible secondary infection.

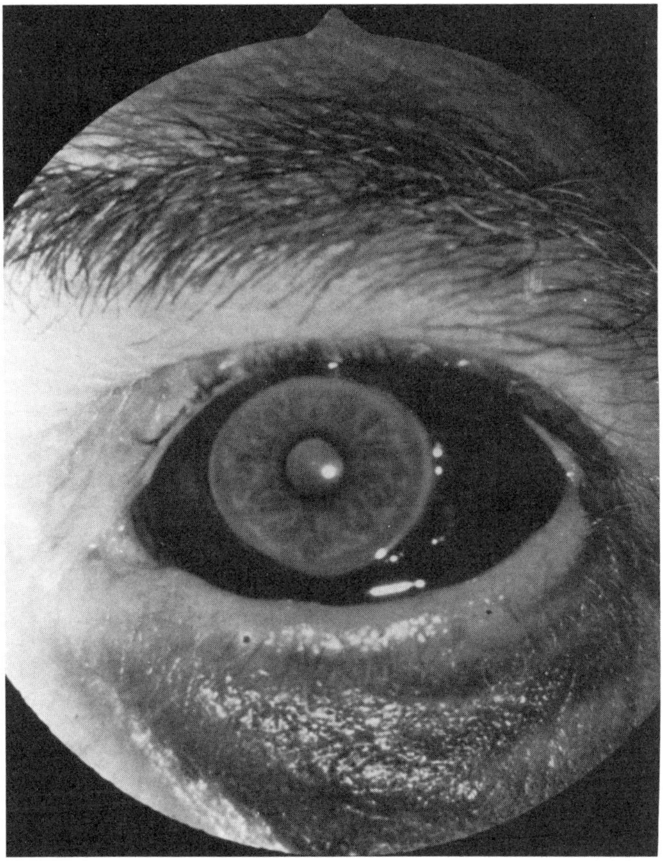

Fig. 5-3. Subconjunctival hemorrhage and ecchymosis of lower lid.

CONTUSION AND CONCUSSION INJURY OF THE CORNEA

Concussion injuries of the cornea may be of two types: concussion necrosis or laceration of tissue.

Direct impact by a blunt object may cause edematous opacities of the corneal epithelium or endothelium. Concussion may cause edematous changes in the substantia propria forming a typically disc-shaped or ring-shaped opacity of 2-3 mm in size. Occasionally, folds of Bowman's or Descemet's membrane, or both, can be observed after a concussion or contusion injury.

A more diffuse and massive edema of the cornea may be seen if the injury causes tears in Descemet's membrane. Very often there is a break in the endothelium layer if the tear occurs in Descemet's membrane. This condition may result in permanent cicatricial opacities. Complete rupture of the entire cornea is extremely rare.

Signs and Symptoms

Pain, photophobia, lacrimation, blepharospasm, and reduced visual acuity might be present in case of a corneal injury due to concussion or contusion.

Treatment

No specific treatment for a concussion or contusion injury of the cornea is available. The routine emergency treatment includes a mild cycloplegic such as Cyclogyl 0. 5%, an antibiotic such as chloromycetin 1%, and patching the eye.

HYPHEMA

Blood in the anterior chamber is called hyphema (Fig. 5-4). The blood may fill the whole anterior chamber or only part of it. If the patient rests in a sitting position, the blood settles in the inferior portion of the anterior chamber. It is important to remember that a patient with hyphema is very often somnolent. Lack of alertness is particularly true in children. The exact mechanism of this somnolence or lethargy is unknown. However, brain concussion or other head injury must be considered also in such a patient, especially when trauma occurs to both the eye and the head.

Treatment

The patient should be relatively still with emphasis on bed rest. The treatment of hyphema is controversial. Since it is a form of traumatic inflammation and iridocyclitis, the treatment is similar.

Local administration of a cycloplegic such as atropine 1% or homatropine 5% is controversial. It provides comfort and decreases the blood-aqueous barrier which reduces the effects of iridocyclitis. Additionally, corticosteroid drops decrease the inflammation. Unilateral or bilateral patching may enhance patient comfort but is also controversial.

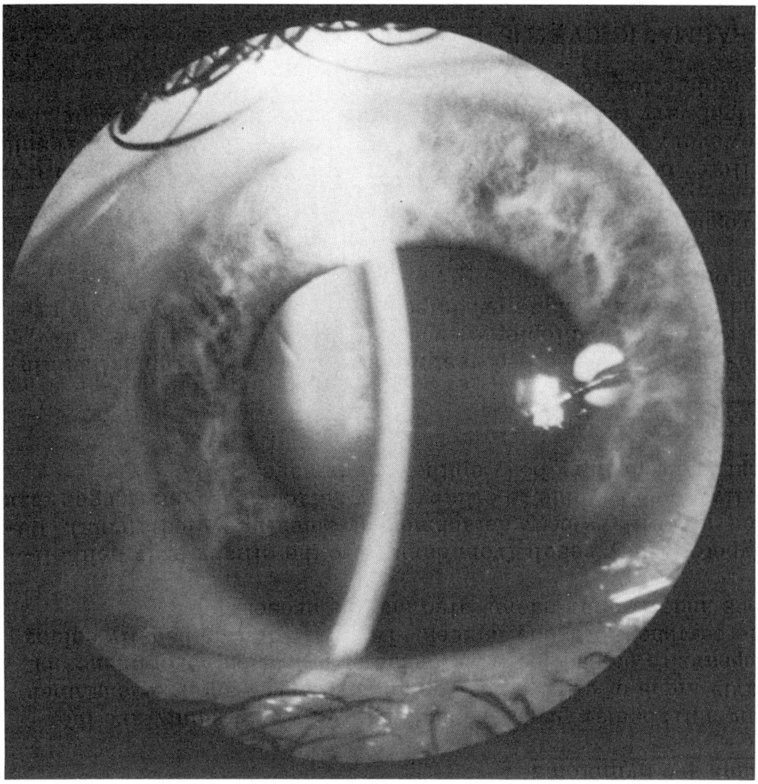

Fig. 5-4. Hyphema covering approximately 10% of the anterior chamber.

An elevated intraocular pressure indicates the presence of secondary glaucoma. It should be treated with topical Timolol 0.5% b.i.d., except when medically contraindicated. Concomitant use of a carbonic anhydrase inhibitor such as Diamox and a hyperosmotic agent such as glycerol may be necessary. The method of administration and the amount of medication to be used are discussed in the chapter on glaucoma.

Late Complications and Their Treatment

Secondary hemorrhage from broken vessels may occur from the third to fifth day following injury. This type of hemorrhage is sometimes more serious than the primary hemorrhage. Secondary glaucoma with severe pain is not an unusual complication.

An eye with hyphema should be examined daily. Long-lasting hyphema may cause blood staining of the cornea. Blood pigment enters the cornea causing a brown discoloration of Descemet's membrane. Corneal staining is most likely to appear if both elevated intraocular pressure and extensive hyphema are present.

Surgical intervention, which means the evacuation of the blood from the anterior chamber, is indicated when either of two conditions obtains: (1) the conservative treatment of secondary glaucoma has proved ineffective, and (2) staining of the cornea is evident.

IRIDODIALYSIS; TRAUMATIC ANIRIDIA; CHANGES IN ACCOMMODATION AND REFRACTION; CHANGES IN THE PUPIL

Iridodialysis (Fig. 5-5) is the disinsertion of the iris from the ciliary body and may occur in association with hyphema or with other pathologic conditions due to blunt trauma. After the initial period of rest no treatment is usually required. Occasionally, the iridodialysis is so extensive that the iris drops down, occluding the visual axis and interfering with useful vision. Diplopia and visual confusion may be present. In these cases, surgical intervention (that is, suturing the iris) is indicated several weeks or months after injury, when the eye is quiet and its condition is stabilized. If the root of the iris is completely torn from its attachment to the ciliary body, the condition is called traumatic aniridia. A complete hyphema usually accompanies this traumatic lesion. After absorption of the blood, a shrunken grey body can be seen in the anterior chamber. Also, complete retroflexion or inversion of the iris may occur in a severe concussion injury. No treatment is indicated in such cases. No medication is effective to correct the deformity.

After blunt trauma, paralysis of the pupil may occur. The pupil may be dilated and may or may not react to light. The accommodation can be impaired as well. This condition, called traumatic mydriasis, may persist for several days, weeks, or occasionally be permanent.

A spastic miosis is an immediate constant sequel to a blunt trauma. The constriction of the pupil is intensive in nature and is usually transient. The exact mechanism of traumatic miosis is not completely understood. In some cases it can be explained as due to sympathetic paralysis resulting from an injury to the skull or neck region.

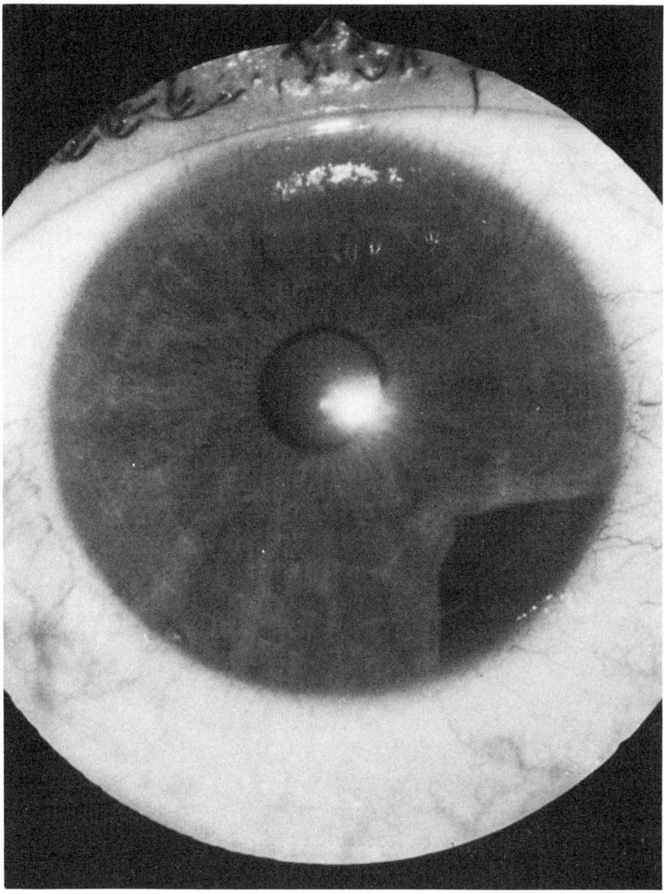

Fig. 5-5. Eye after trauma. Iridodialysis is seen nasally. The lens is cataractous.

Sometimes the pupil is irregular after trauma, due to rupture of the sphincter muscle of the iris. Irregularity of the pupil may be temporary or it may be permanent, lasting for the patient's lifetime. Trauma to the eye is usually followed by inflammation of the uveal tissue. Traumatic anterior uveitis also causes constriction of the pupil. After a blunt trauma, changes in the refraction may occur. Transient hypermetropia or myopia may occur.

CILIARY BODY DETACHMENT

Dysfunction of the ciliary body following concussion injury is not an uncommon complication.

Signs and Symptoms

Low intraocular pressure and reduced visual acuity are the early signs of ciliary body detachment. The anterior chamber appears to be shallow. On fundus examination, prominence of the peripheral fundus is seen. The optic disc is usually edematous and macular edema also may be present.

Hypotony may result from damage to the ciliary body epithelium, and ciliary body detachment (traumatic cyclodialysis). Usually, hypotony due to ciliary body detachment lasts longer than that due to ciliary body epithelium damage.

Treatment

Hospitalization and bed rest may be necessary. Topical administration of a cycloplegic such as Cyclogyl 1%, 3 times a day, and a steroid such as prednisone 30-60 mg a day by mouth are recommended.

Prognosis

Ciliary body detachment following trauma is usually temporary; however, it may last for weeks or even months. The end result might vary from complete recovery to severe glaucoma or complete loss of function of the affected eye.

TRAUMATIC UVEITIS

Traumatic uveitis is a very common condition. It may occur in any contusion injury or after severe corneal injury including foreign body, laceration, or chemical injury, and is more severe in a heavily pigmented eye. Traumatic uveitis may not be present immediately after injury, but it may appear a few hours or days after the injury.

Signs and Symptoms

The patient's visual acuity is reduced. Photophobia is common and often severe. The patient suffers from pain of the affected eye, headache also may occur, the conjunctiva is red, the episcleral vessels are engorged, and the pupil is constricted.

Treatment

Obviously, if a causative agent is responsible, it should be removed. A short-acting cycloplegic, such as cyclopentolate 0.5% (Cyclogyl) and a mydriatic (Neosynephrine 10%) should be administered. If the uveitis is severe, the drops should be used 3-4 times a day. Dark glasses or patching of the affected eye help to relieve the discomfort. Topical steroid drops also should be considered in the event that the corneal epithelium is intact and there is no sign of bacterial or fungal infection.

RECESSION OF THE ANTERIOR CHAMBER ANGLE AND OTHER CONDITIONS CAUSING GLAUCOMA

The effect of a concussion or a contusion injury on the intraocular pressure may be dramatic and sometimes a determining factor concerning the fate of the eye. The rise in tension usually develops immediately or shortly after the injury. In 20% of cases it may develop more than 1 week later. The cause of concussion glaucoma is not well understood. It may be complex and not necessarily an injury to one particular part of the eye.

Recession of the anterior chamber angle has been mentioned as a common cause of posttraumatic elevated intraocular pressure. Biomicroscopic examination of these cases shows areas with a wide open angle of the anterior chamber. It is believed to be due to displacement of certain structures, such as the ciliary muscles, from the trabecular meshwork area. In addition to these macroscopic changes, the normal histology of the trabecular meshwork and the whole drainage system are injured as well. The rise in intraocular pressure may occur years after the injury.

Thrombosis of ciliary veins and endothelial changes in the vortex veins are also among the possibilities which can cause elevated intraocular pressure after contusion or concussion injury. Subluxation or dislocation of the lens, herniation of the vitreous, and intraocular hemorrhages are responsible in different ways for elevated intraocular pressure after trauma. These conditions are discussed elsewhere in this chapter.

Treatment

Initial treatment of concussion glaucoma is not different from other types of secondary glaucoma. To reduce intraocular pressure, carbonic anhydrase inhibitors and hyperosmotic agents can be used immediately after diagnosis. Diamox 250 mg, 4 times a day by mouth, or glycerol 1 g/kg body weight, 2-3 times a day, might be effective to reduce intraocular pressure. In addition to the above, miotic eyedrops such as pilocarpine 2% should be administered 3-4 times a day. Occasionally, sympathomimetic eyedrops such as epinephrine or norepinephrine 1% (Eppy 1%), administered twice a day helps to reduce the intraocular pressure. Timolol 0.5% used twice daily is also effective in these cases.

TRAUMATIC CATARACT; TRAUMATIC DISLOCATION OF THE LENS; HERNIATION OF THE VITREOUS INTO THE ANTERIOR CHAMBER

Cataract development after contusion of the eyeball is not unusual and may occur without any detectable damage to the capsule. The exact mechanism of this type of cataract is not known. Generally, the cataract must be extracted several months after injury if optically disabling.

Blunt trauma to the eyeball can cause subluxation or complete luxation of the lens (see Fig. 5-6). The striking force tears the zonules holding the lens in place behind the iris in the center of the pupil. If the lens drops into the vitreous body, the condition is called complete dislocation of the lens. If part of the zonules remain intact, the lens is pulled slightly toward the intact zonules. This condition is called subluxation of the lens.

The anterior chamber may deepen in these conditions and iridodonesis (trembling of the iris) also can be seen. The hyaloid face of the vitreous may be disturbed and the vitreous may herniate into the anterior chamber. Occasionally, the lens may become partly or completely dislocated into the anterior chamber. This situation may cause a shallow anterior chamber. Also, the lens may touch the posterior surface of the cornea. Very often, secondary glaucoma accompanies these conditions. The most common mechanism of secondary glaucoma is pupillary block. The aqueous cannot pass from the posterior chamber through the pupil into the anterior chamber because the lens, or the vitreous, occludes the pupil completely or partially.

Treatment

When dislocation of the lens or herniation of the vitreous causes an elevated intraocular pressure, immediate surgical

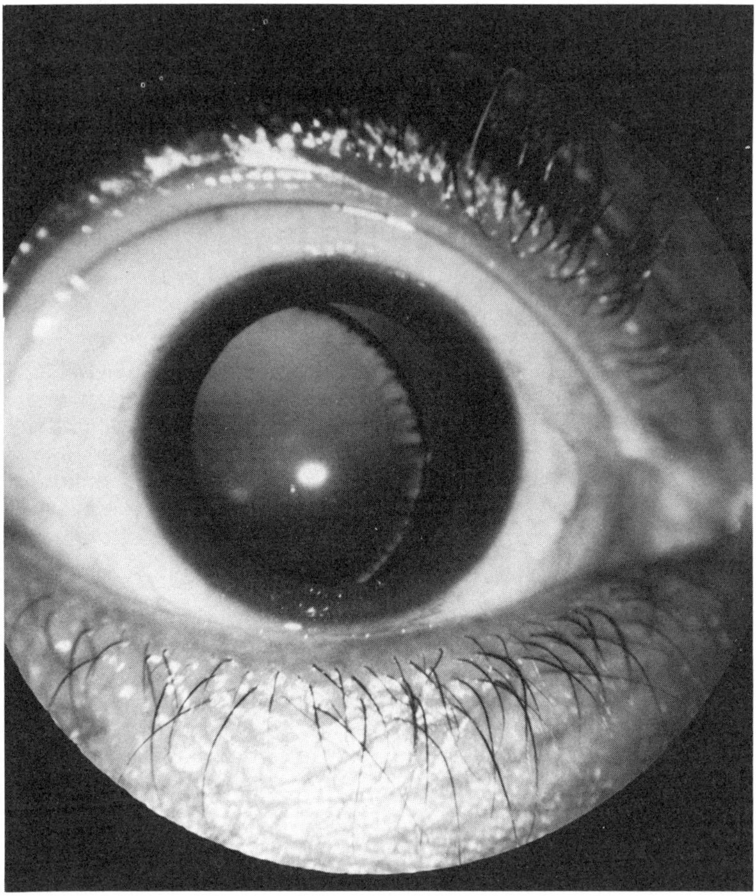

Fig. 5-6. Traumatic subluxated lens.

intervention is not indicated. The secondary glaucoma should be treated. The condition of the eye should be completely evaluated, including visual acuity, intraocular pressure, and other pathologic conditions caused by the trauma. In general, complete dislocation of the lens into the vitreous cavity rarely requires lens extraction. If the lens is partly dislocated and occludes the pupil, causing secondary glaucoma, laser surgery is indicated. Laser therapy can create iridotomies in the iris periphery to provide alternate pathways for the aqueous to flow. Laser therapy is very successful and further conventional surgical intervention may be avoided. Herniation of the vitreous through the pupil causes elevated intraocular pressure and also calls for laser surgery. Lens extraction combined with anterior vitrectomy may be required for visual rehabilitation. This surgical intervention should be performed electively after the ocular inflammation has subsided. Complete dislocation of the lens into the anterior chamber will cause corneal decompensation as well as secondary glaucoma. Surgical extraction is immediately indicated.

VITREOUS HEMORRHAGE

Vitreous hemorrhage caused by trauma is a serious condition. The hemorrhage may originate from retinal vessels or from the uvea. The route of absorption, damage to different ocular tissues, and the early and late complications after vitreous hemorrhage are discussed in more detail in Chapter 2 under the section entitled "Vitreous Hemorrhage."

Signs and Symptoms

If no other pathologic condition accompanies vitreous hemorrhage there is little, if any, pathology present in the anterior segment of the eye. The pupil may be more dilated in the affected eye than in the fellow eye. The patient's visual acuity is markedly decreased, sometimes reduced to light perception only. On fundus examination, no details of the fundus can be seen because of vitreous haze. Occasionally, the vitreous hemorrhage is so severe that the red reflex of the fundus cannot be elicited. On examination, the reflex is black.

Treatment

There is no specific treatment for vitreous hemorrhage. Rest in a sitting position may be helpful because the blood cells will gravitate to the lower part of the vitreous and, in this way, the central portion of the vitreous body will clear up sooner. Bilateral patching is useful; however, if the patient is restless with both eyes occluded, it is considered best to abandon the bilateral patching. The effectiveness of an oral or a subconjunctival enzymatic agent such as Varidase (streptokynase and streptodornase enzymes), fibrinolysin, or Chymolase (pancreatic enzyme) is questionable.

Mechanical removal of opaque vitreous, that is, partial or total vitrectomy, is advocated by many ophthalmic surgeons. This may be considered only if the absorption of blood has been insufficient after a period of a few months.

Prognosis

The patient may resume his usual activities a few weeks after injury but vigorous motion of the head and eyes must be avoided. Absorption of blood from the vitreous body may take many weeks or months. Occasionally, the blood may organize in the vitreous causing retinal detachment and serious loss of visual acuity.

RUPTURE OF THE CHOROID

Severe contusion or concussion injury of the eyeball can cause rupture of the choroid. At the time of injury only vitreous or retinal hemorrhage can be seen, with marked deterioration of vision. After absorption of the hemorrhage a whitish, semicircular scar with mild pigmentation can be seen at the posterior pole (Fig. 5-7). In more than four-fifths of the cases, the fissures are on the temporal side of the disc. A nasal crescent is rare and horizontal ruptures are seen only occasionally. If the whitish scar transects the papillomacular nerve bundles (the nerve fibers between the optic disc and the macular area), the resulting visual acuity is always poor (20/200-20/400). Occasionally, the scar is outside the macular area and causes only minor changes in visual acuity but does cause a visual field defect. The only treatment required is bed rest for a few days after injury.

Choroidal Hemorrhage

Hemorrhage of the choroid is a relatively common sequel to contusion injury and may occur without rupture of the Bruch's membrane or the layer of the pigment epithelium. The hemorrhage can spread between the choroid and the sclera, detaching the choroid from the sclera. On fundus examination, the area of choroidal hemorrhage seems to be elevated and has a dark brown color. The vision may or may not be affected, depending on the site and extent of the damage. No immediate effective treatment is known for choroidal hemorrhage. Bed rest, with the head elevated, for several days, is the conventional treatment.

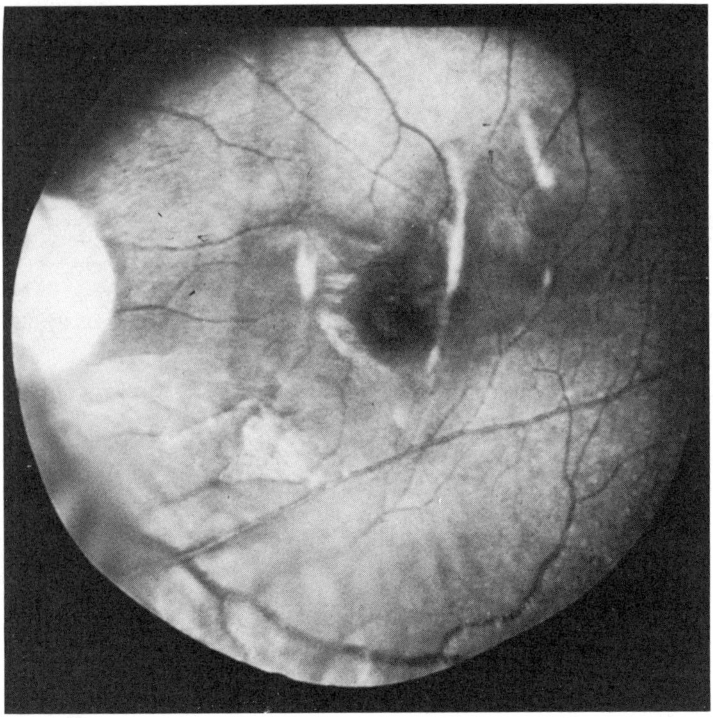

Fig. 5-7. Rupture of the choroid.

Chorioretinal Rupture

Occasionally, a simultaneous rupture of both the choroid and the retina may occur. If the retina also is torn, the hemorrhage may extend into the vitreous. This type of injury is more common in war when the striking force is great. At the time of injury the fundus rarely can be seen. Later, proliferating chorioretinitis, originating from the site of injury, often causes retinal detachment by traction.

Traumatic Choroiditis

Traumatic injuries may occur in blast injuries. It is believed that first the striking force causes tissue necrosis. The necrotic tissue initiates vascular reaction which causes hemorrhage. Considerable degrees of pigment proliferation and subsequent atrophy of the uveal tissue is the usual course.

The symptoms of traumatic choroiditis are the same as those of mechanical rupture of the choroid. The treatment is the same as in choroidal rupture, that is, bed rest for a few days.

RETINAL HEMORRHAGE AND EDEMA

Shortly after injury, hemorrhage or edema may be found in the retina. Hemorrhages can be subhyaloid, preretinal, in the superficial layers of the retina, or in the deeper layers of the retina. The more anterior the retinal hemorrhage, the brighter is the red color. Deep hemorrhages are rather greyish or bluish-red. The hemorrhages may occur in different shapes depending on the depth (Fig. 5-8). Round hemorrhages are located deep in the retina, while flame-shaped hemorrhages are more superficial.

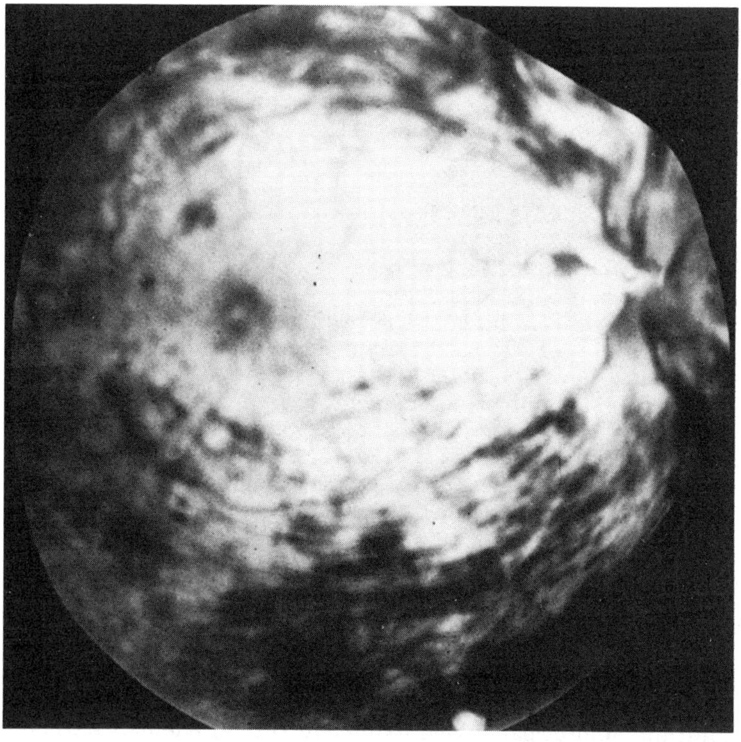

Fig. 5-8. Retinal hemorrhages after contusion injury of the eyeball.

Edema of the retina may appear at the site of the injury or, more commonly, at the posterior pole. This condition is called Berlin's edema or commotio retinae.

Despite the retinal hemorrhages, the visual acuity can remain very good unless the hemorrhage occurs in the macular area. Edema of the retina, especially edema at the posterior pole, causes reduced visual acuity. The prognosis of retinal hemorrhage and edema is unpredictable. In certain cases the edema or the hemorrhage, or both, absorb quickly with no significant damage to the vision. In other cases the edema disappears weeks after the injury; in these cases, the visual acuity may be markedly reduced.

Treatment

No specific treatment is known for retinal hemorrhage or retinal edema. If the retinal edema persists for longer periods of time with no sign of improvement, oral steroid treatment might be beneficial. Many ophthalmologists treat retinal edema with high doses of steroid (prednisone 120 mg/day) immediately after the injury.

TRAUMATIC RETINAL DETACHMENT

There are two main groups of detachments to be considered concerning trauma. In one group, a retinal hole or disinsertion occurs at the time of injury. These holes, or disinsertions, are responsible for retinal detachment at a later stage. In the other group, there are no holes in the retina at the time of injury. Vitreous hemorrhage occurs and, later, the vitreous hemorrhage leads to traction band formation in the vitreous body. These traction bands pull on the retina, either tearing it or detaching it. Other conditions which may cause retinal detachment are retinal edema and hemorrhage. The retina becomes necrotic and cystic in those areas with the edema or hemorrhage and finally retinal holes develop. These holes occasionally may cause retinal detachment at a later stage (Fig. 5-9).

In most cases of contusion or concussion of the eye the prominent ophthalmoscopic appearance of the fundus is the presence of multiple hemorrhages and extensive retinal edema. Retinal tears can be seen only occasionally. Most of the holes or tears are peripheral to the equator and are not visible with a direct ophthalmoscope. It is difficult to differentiate between areas of severe retinal edema and retinal detachment occurring immediately or shortly after the initial trauma.

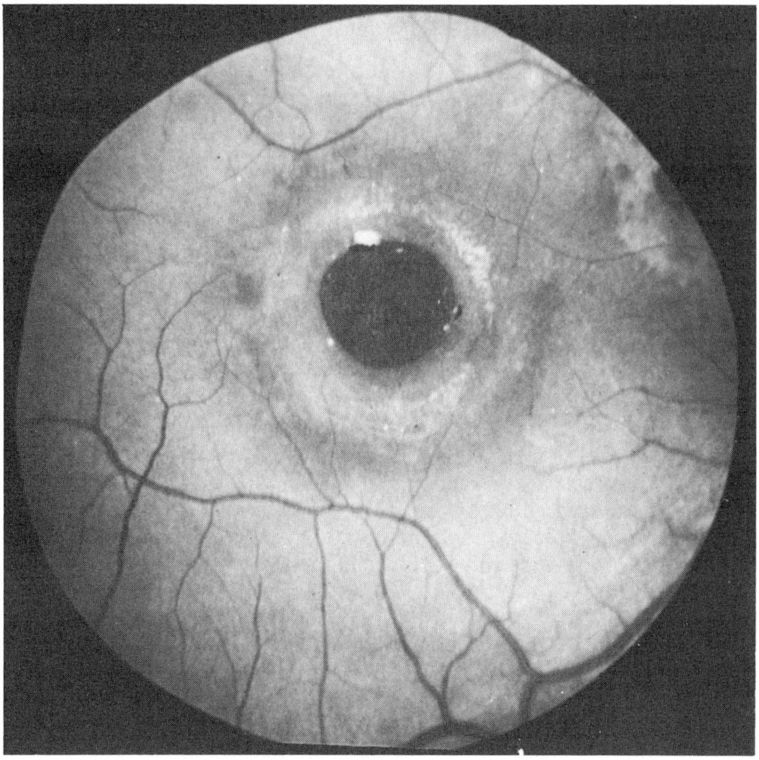

Fig. 5-9. Retinal hole of traumatic origin at the macula. The retina is detached around the hole.

Treatment

Traumatic retinal detachment should be treated differently from other types of detachment. Immediate surgery may not be indicated. Bed rest and careful reexamination and reevaluation by an ophthalmologist should be an almost routine requirement. The emergency room physician should instruct the patient to undergo such an examination. Ophthalmic ultrasonography is an invaluable tool for confirming retinal detachments especially when a cloudy media is present.

RUPTURE OF THE EYEBALL

Rupture of the eyeball due to blunt trauma occurs quite often. The signs, symptoms, and management of the ruptured globe will be discussed in Chapter 6.

RETINOPATHY DUE TO DISTANCE INJURY (PURTSCHER'S DISEASE)

A patient involved in a car accident or suffering from head or chest injury may present with a special type of retinopathy which is called Purtscher's disease or "angiopathia retinae traumatica." The eyes are not involved directly in the accident and, except for the retina, do not show much pathology. The pathogenesis of the disease is not known. Purtscher explains the changes in the retina to be caused by "pronounced rise in the pressure of the cerebrospinal fluid, which is transmitted to the perivascular lymph space of the central vessels in the optic nerve. This pressure mechanism causes the escape of blood cells and plasma into the retinal tissue."

SIGNS AND SYMPTOMS

The condition appears within the first 2 days after injury. The visual acuity may or may not be impaired, depending on the degree of involvement of the macular area. The eye shows minimal pathologic damage except in the retina. On fundus examination, superficial round, white, patchy exudates are seen close to the retinal veins. Small linear hemorrhages can be seen all around the posterior pole. Edema of the perimacular area is common. In general, the arteries are narrow and the veins are congested.

TREATMENT

No treatment is available.

PROGNOSIS

The fundus changes gradually disappear within a few days or weeks. The vision may or may not return to normal, depending on how severely the macular area was involved.

LATE COMPLICATIONS AFTER BLUNT TRAUMA TO THE EYEBALL

PHACOLYTIC GLAUCOMA

A lens which has been traumatized can develop a cataract. Occasionally, the cataract may be hypermature. The cortical material of the lens becomes liquified and leaks through the lens capsule into the anterior chamber. This lens material flares up into a characteristic macrophage reaction in the anterior segment of the eye. Proteinaceous material and cellular debris clog the outflow channels of the aqueous humor. This condition, the combination of severe anterior uveitis and extremely high intraocular tension, is called phacolytic glaucoma. Phacolytic glaucoma may occur also without any history of trauma.

Signs and Symptoms

The patient suffers from severe eye and head pain. The vision might be light perception only. The intraocular pressure is high and the cornea is hazy. The eye has a congested appearance because of engorged conjunctival vessels. If the anterior chamber can be seen through the cornea, severe flare and a large number of cells can be observed and a cataractous lens is seen behind the constricted pupil.

Treatment

Phacolytic glaucoma is one of the rare conditions when emergency cataract extraction is indicated. Conservative treatment does not improve the condition of the eye and the high intraocular pressure may cause permanent blindness within a short period of time. The intraocular pressure must be reduced by a hyperosmotic agent such as intravenous mannitol.

Prognosis

The postoperative course is benign in most cases. The inflammation subsides quickly and the intraocular pressure returns to normal. Visual acuity may vary between useful vision and light perception, depending on how long the intraocular pressure was elevated and how much of the optic nerve was damaged.

BIBLIOGRAPHY

Bibliography for this chapter is included at the end of Chapter 6, Trauma: Part II.

Chapter 6

TRAUMA: PART II – PENETRATING AND PERFORATING INJURIES OF THE EYEBALL

Penetrating or perforating ocular injuries are very serious injuries that may result in loss of vision. Violence (knives and glass) and industrial accidents (steel bits, stone fragments) accounted for 55% of all penetrating injuries in a series from the Newark Eye and Ear Infirmary. Etiology can vary among socioeconomic populations. Children's toys (darts, arrows), automobile accidents, and domestic injuries account for another 25% of serious injuries.

The location of the penetration and the extent of ocular tissue damage will determine the prognosis of these injuries. Emergency care is also vital to protect the existing integrity of the eye.

The following procedure is indicated, regardless of whether or not the wound is large or small or the clinical picture is complicated by prolapse of intraocular content:

1. History
2. Eye examination
3. Ultrasonography
4. X-ray examination
5. Tetanus prophylaxis and antibiotic therapy
6. Surgical intervention (if necessary)

1. History of the injury: A complete history of the accident should be obtained. In determining the seriousness of the

injury, the details of the occurrence are invaluable. If a projectile is involved an attempt should be made to obtain a sample of this projectile. In the case of metal, it is imperative to test for magnetic properties. If the material is glass, then its lead content may show radiolucency.

2. Examination of the eyeball requires careful examination. No pressure should be applied to the globe when a penetrating or perforating injury is suspected. Minimal eye examination should include vision, examination of the lids and adnexae, examination of the anterior segment, and at least an attempt to examine the posterior segment. If the examination is painful, or if it might endanger the integrity of the globe (as in the case of a large wound), the extent of the injury should be evaluated as best as possible without manipulation.

   Under no circumstances should visual acuity examination be neglected, especially for medicolegal reasons. In many cases, it is impossible to have the patient stand 20 feet from a Snellen chart. Any objects with print (e. g. , newspaper, matchcover, typewritten letters) should be held with each eye alternately occluded. Any vision should be noted. For example, "patient able to read headline of newspaper." The ability of the patient to see fingers may be noted also, e. g. , "patient can count fingers at 5 feet." This record can have important influence on the treatment of the injury. Pupillary reflexes should be noted in all cases.

3. Ultrasonography: All eyes with severe penetrating or perforating injuries should have ocular ultrasound to determine if any intraocular foreign bodies are present and to evaluate the extent of the injury (the degree of disorganization of the retina and vitreous). The ultrasound should be performed by an experienced ophthalmologist to prevent further damage to the eye from the examination.

4. X-ray examination of the injured eye is necessary to determine the presence and location of a radiopaque intraocular foreign body. This examination is described in detail in the chapter on Emergency Ophthalmologic Radiology.

5. Tetanus prophylaxis should be given in the emergency room.

6. Antibiotic therapy should be started prophylactically. If hospitalization or surgery is planned, an intravenous should be started and a broad spectrum antibiotic administered.

7. Surgical intervention: Successful surgical intervention and the possibility of preserving the useful function of the eye are often possible. The need for surgery can be determined only by an ophthalmologist.

TERMINOLOGY AND CLASSIFICATION OF PENETRATING AND PERFORATING EYE INJURIES

Penetrating injury refers to partial tissue damage of the outer coat of the eye (cornea or sclera). An example of this injury is when a foreign body with low velocity enters into the sclera and remains impacted among the lamellae, or a sharp object cuts through two-thirds of the cornea leaving Descemet's membrane intact. This type of injury is not a true through-and-through wound of the sclera or cornea.

Perforating injury refers to complete discontinuation of tissue through the entire thickness of the coat of the eyeball; in other words, an open wound is present through the cornea or the sclera. Perforating injury can be divided into three groups:

1. Perforating injury without retained intraocular foreign body
2. Perforating injury with retained intraocular foreign body
3. Double perforation of the globe (Fig. 6-1)

The term laceration also is used commonly, especially when a through-and-through corneal (or scleral) wound is present.

SIGNS OF PERFORATION OF THE EYEBALL

The following signs may be indicative of perforation of the globe:

1. Reduced visual acuity
2. Reduced intraocular pressure (hypotony)
3. Change in depth of the anterior chamber
4. Displacement of the pupil or change in the shape of the pupil
5. Visible would of the cornea or the sclera
6. Prolapse of ocular tissue (uvea, lens, vitreous, retina)
7. Chemosis of the conjunctiva (edema)

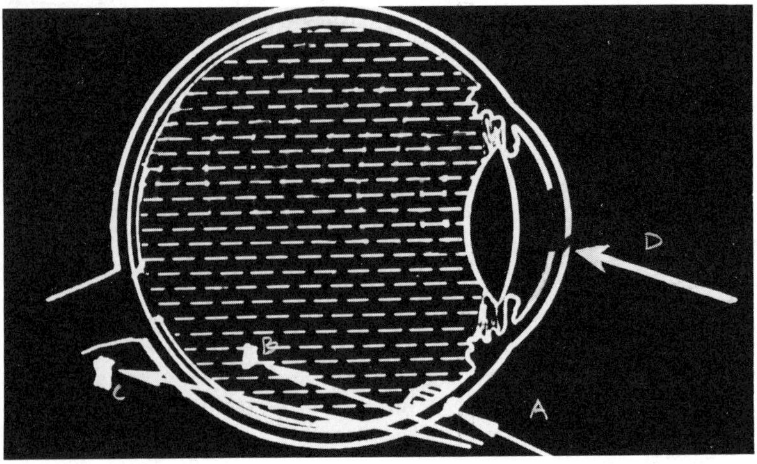

Fig. 6-1. Artist's drawing, A) penetrating injury to the sclera. A foreign body is impacted among the scleral lamellae; B) perforating injury with retained intraocular foreign body; C) double perforation with a foreign particle; D) corneal perforation.

In the case of a perforation, not all of the above-mentioned signs are always present. On the other hand, these signs are not pathognomonic for perforating injury, but may occur in other conditions. For example, low intraocular pressure may present after blunt trauma to the eye with no perforation. Also, chemosis of the conjunctiva may occur in many conditions with no perforation of the globe.

The depth of the anterior chamber changes in almost all cases of perforated injury. It becomes shallow if the perforation is in the anterior segment, since the aqueous humor escapes through the perforation. The anterior chamber becomes deep if the perforation is posterior and ocular tissue protrudes through the wound.

The pupil can change its shape and position if anterior uveal tissue (iris, ciliary body) extrudes through the wound, whether or not the wound is visible. A perforation should always be suspected in such cases.

IMMEDIATE MANAGEMENT OF PENETRATING OR PERFORATING INJURY

Life-saving measures have priority over eye care; however, immediate minimal care of a penetrating or perforating injury of the eye may not interfere with life-saving measures and, therefore, should not be neglected or unduly postponed.

The injured eye should be treated in the emergency room after thorough and careful examination, as already described in this chapter. The treatment can be divided into two parts: general and supportive therapy and ocular treatment.

The general and supportive therapy should include massive antibiotic treatment, corticosteroids, tetanus prophylaxis, analgesics, sedation, and antiemetic, if necessary. All medications should be administered intramuscularly or intravenously. Oral intake of food or beverages should be discontinued immediately. These measures will permit the patient to be anesthetized safely for surgical repair when optimal conditions for surgery are present. Nausea or vomiting should be suppressed by proper medication, as vomiting increases the intraocular pressure which may result in unnecessary prolapse of intraocular tissue through the open wound; also, it might cause hemorrhage from the damaged tissue. The physhologic effect of an eye injury also should be considered; the patient should be adequately sedated until the damaged globe can be repaired.

Topical treatment of the injured eye in the emergency room should be minimal. Instillation of antibiotic eyedrops such as Chloroptic (chloromycetin 0.5%), Garamycin, or Neosporin, and patching of the eye are essential. A single eye patch with an ophthalmic shield should be used. However, mydriatic or miotic eyedrops should not be used prior to surgery as the effect of these medications might make the necessary surgical repair more difficult. The use of any kind of ointment is not recommended when an open wound is present, as it might penetrate the open globe.

TYPES OF INJURIES

Anterior segment injuries vary from simple nonpenetrating corneal lacerations to complete avulsion of and destruction of the anterior globe. We shall begin with a simple outline of the various types of injuries and then proceed with suggestions for their repair.

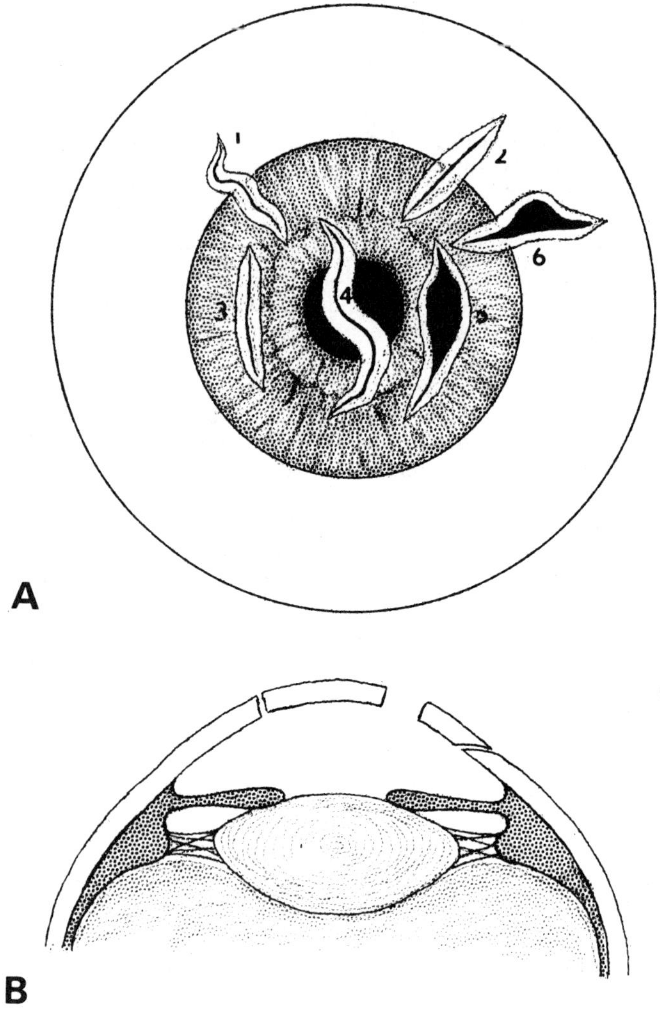

Fig. 6-2A and B. (A) Diagrammatic representation of corneal and corneoscleral lacerations: 1) irregular corneoscleral laceration; 2) linear corneoscleral laceration; 3) linear corneal laceration; 4) irregular corneal laceration; 5) avulsing corneal laceration; 6) avulsing corneoscleral laceration. (B) Diagrammatic representation of vertical, oblique, and avulsing corneal lacerations.

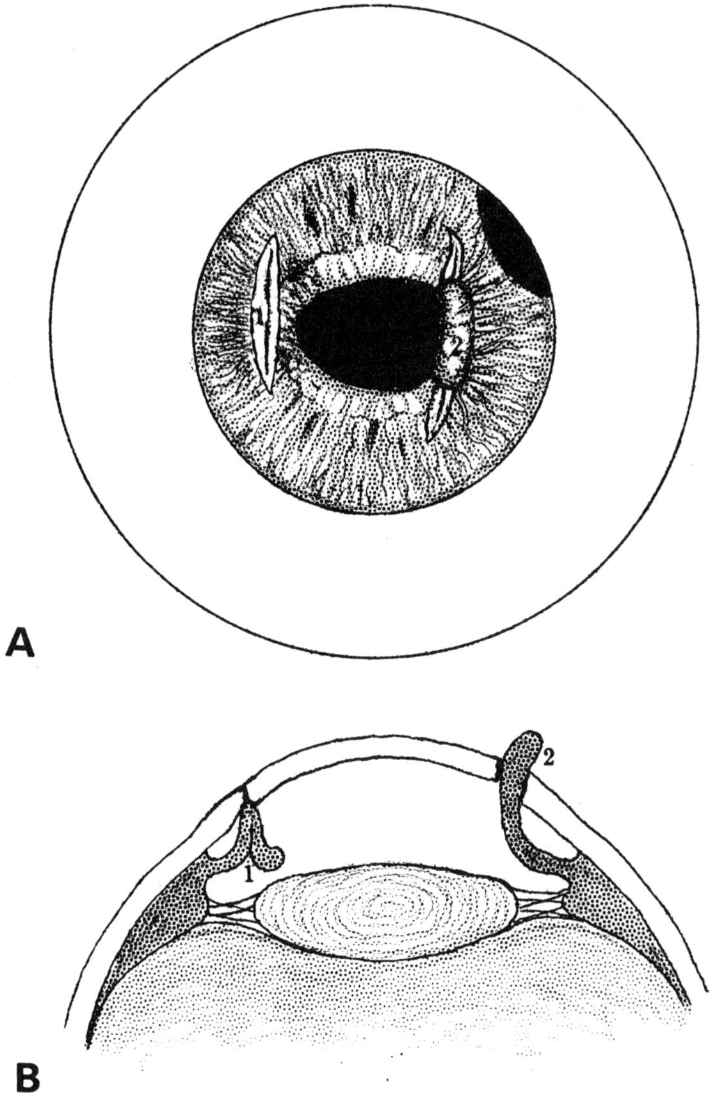

Figs. 6-3A and B. Diagrammatic representation of a penetrating laceration with iris incarceration: (1) left, entirely internal; (2) right, iris prolapsed externally.

CORNEAL LACERATIONS

Simple corneal laceration (Fig. 6-2A) can be linear, irregular, or avulsing with the lacerating implement entering either vertically or obliquely (Fig. 6-2B) in a particular injury. The incision may be partially penetrating or penetrating, or both. The anterior segment may be otherwise unharmed or the penetrating laceration may involve the iris. This latter can be either entirely internal (Figs. 6-3A and B) or prolapsed externally (Figs. 6-3A and B) with or without iris laceration. When incarcerated, iris sphincter or the dilator fibers, or both, can be included in the wound. It is evident that the more central the lesion, the less likely for peripheral iris to be prolapsed, and vice versa.

Peripheral iris injuries are more liable to be lacerating because of the closer proximity of the iris to the cornea. In addition, they are more difficult to disengage from corneal laceration and more likely to form postoperative anterior synechiae even if apparently effectively released at surgery. If a simple incarceration of nonlacerated iris is seen immediately and there are no attendant generalized injuries preventing immediate repair, this can be considered an eye surgical emergency. The immediate repositioning of the iris with suturing of the corneal laceration can prevent iris necrosis. Delayed surgical repair makes reposition difficult or impossible as prolonged incarceration may produce sphincter or dilator paralysis and an irregular pupil.

Corneal laceration may be complicated also by an accompanying disruption of the lens (Figs. 6-4A and B). If this occurs without iris involvement there is usually disruption of the anterior capsule only. A point-penetrating injury such as that caused by a wire may go through-and-through the lens (Fig. 6-4B), even to pierce the posterior globe, finally to enter the posterior orbit.

The more peripheral the corneal lesion and iris trauma, the greater the likelihood that hemorrhage will accompany such compound injuries to the anterior segment. The extent of posterior injury can be completely obscured by blood and the laceration and its attendant posterior damage can be thoroughly evaluated and managed only at surgery.

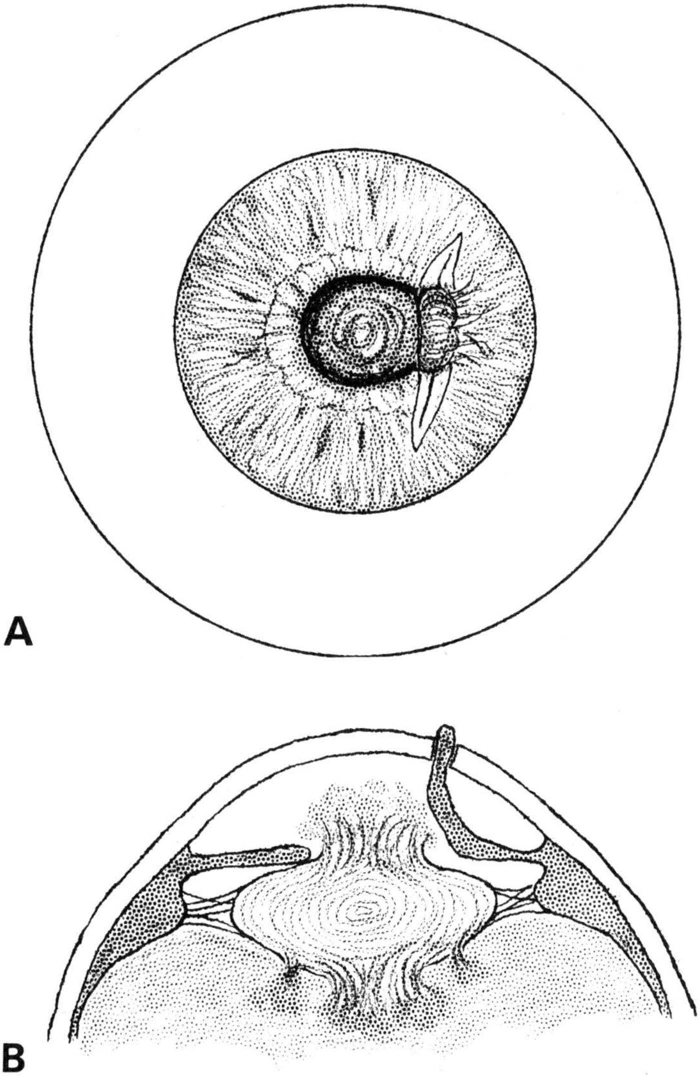

Figs. 6-4A and B. Diagrammatic representation of corneal laceration with iris prolapse and disruption of the lens. (A) anterior view; (B) cross-section.

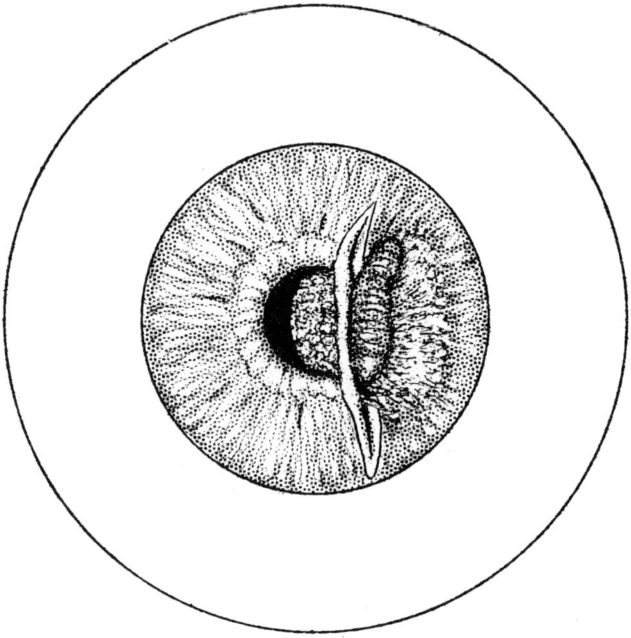

A

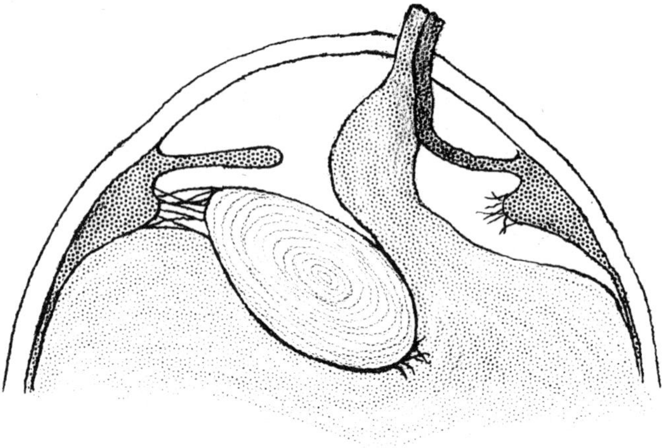

B

Figs. 6-5A and B. Diagrammatic representation of corneal laceration with prolapse of iris and vitreous and dislocated lens. (A) anterior view; (B) cross-section.

LENS INJURIES

The lens may be dislocated without being lacerated (Fig. 6-5B) or both with disruption of the anterior and, sometimes, the posterior capsule. Lens dislocation in the young patient is rare, but the older the patient, the weaker the zonular attachments to the lens, and lens dislocation may be seen more frequently. Vitreous then prolapses forward to become involved with the iris in the anterior laceration (Figs. 6-5A and B). In the case of through-and-through penetration of the lens, with or without dislocation, vitreous is involved and may be seen often in the anterior segment or protruding through the wound with the lens material. In a laceration such as this, if the iris is involved, the traumatic penetration of the lens, when it is small, is sometimes obscured by the iris injury and may be missed by the surgeon even when operating under microscope magnification. The postoperative development of cataract, of course, indicates that lens trauma actually had occurred and was overlooked. However, in a doubtful situation, the later management of a delayed developing traumatic cataract with an apparently intact capsule is preferable to immediate lens removal.

In rare instances the escape of lens material may produce an anaphylactic reaction causing severe granulomatous uveitis. Lens material may also clog the trabecular spaces producing secondary glaucoma. Therefore, during surgical procedure, complete removal of the nucleus and cortex, when indicated, will give a better prognosis.

SCLERAL LACERATIONS

Lacerations involving the anterior sclera can be simple or, as is the usual case, combined with corneal laceration (Fig. 6-2 A). They, too, may be linear, irregular, or avulsing with through-and-through or partial penetration entering vertically or obliquely (Fig. 6-2B). Because of its juxtaposition to the anterior scleral coat, the highly vascular ciliary body is almost invariably involved in anterior scleral lacerations and, as is the case with very peripheral penetrating injuries of the cornea, hemorrhage is the rule rather than the exception. Though laceration of the vitreous with presentation of vitreous through the wound is a common accompaniment of scleral injuries, traumatic damage to the lens is less frequent. Indeed, the globe may be partially, or even completely, collapsed as a result of vitreous loss through a scleral laceration and the lens can remain intact. Injuries posterior to the ciliary body and the pars plana differ somewhat from a wound in the anterior segment because of the presence of the retina behind the ora serrata. These, however, may be merely extensions of anterior injuries. As a general rule, the more posterior the injury, the less chance for survival of vision, since complications involving the retina and vitreous tend to be more severe and less responsive to medical and surgical therapy.

Management

It should be reemphasized that, in most instances, the definitive repair of a lacerating injury to the anterior segment or posterior segment is not an absolute emergency procedure. In an instance when severe general injuries threaten the patient's life, these must be dealt with first. When possible, repair of the eye injuries should be delayed to permit the use of general anesthesia so that a careful and complete primary repair can be performed. However, if at all possible, repair should be effected within the first 24 hours after the injury and no later than 48 hours after the injury. The deeper and more extensive the eye injury, the greater the posttraumatic inflammatory reaction and the greater the possibility of infection. Early debridement and repair will help to reduce the extensive inflammation and severe infection which can result from prolonged retention of damaged or necrotic tissue or infectious agents introduced at the time of injury. Since antibiotics and steroids take some hours to have their full effect, reparative surgery is best performed when antibiotic and antisuppressive therapy has reached its highest therapeutic level, 24-48 hours after injury. Microsurgical technique using fine instrumentation and nonreacting monofilament sutures should be used to minimize surgical trauma and to remove substances which might provoke scarring. Thus, an air- and water-tight wound can be achieved, which might prevent the later complications of scarring, adhesions and/or contraction. Repair of anterior lacerations must restore the anterior chamber to the most physiological state possible, free of vitreous and blood, which can stimulate fibrosis and close the angle. Repair of deeper injuries may also require vitrectomy.

INTRAOCULAR FOREIGN BODIES

The retention of a foreign body within the eye is not a very common injury. However, an intraocular foreign body should be

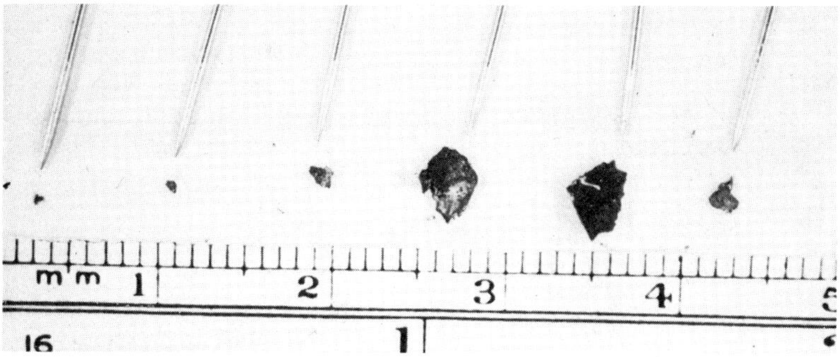

Fig. 6-6. Metallic foreign bodies of different size removed from a patient's eyes.

suspected if periorbital or ocular tissue damage or wounds are visible. The emergency room physician must rule out the presence of an intraocular foreign body in each case, regardless of the patient's history concerning the injury. Intraocular foreign bodies can be divided into two main groups: metallic foreign bodies and nonmetallic foreign bodies. Metallic foreign bodies can be further subdivided into magnetic and nonmagnetic foreign bodies. Both metallic and nonmetallic foreign bodies include inert substances which cause very little, if any, reaction within the eye. Such inert substances include gold, silver, platinum, or tantalum. Nonmetallic inert substances are stone, glass, porcelain, carbon, and certain plastics. An irritative material can be either metallic or nonmetallic. Metallic materials are lead, zinc, nickel, aluminum, copper, and iron (Fig. 6-6). There are many irritative nonmetallic substances, including vegetables, cloth particles, cilia, and eyelid particles.

The eye reacts to a retained foreign body in various ways, depending on the composition of the particle. Some are inert for an indefinite period of time, while others may enter into chemical combination with the tissue and cause severe reaction. The same type of foreign body may react differently in different ocular tissues. In general, a foreign body in the anterior chamber or in the lens causes much less reaction than does one in the posterior segment. The ocular reaction may be of three types:

1. Certain nonorganized material causes no specific reaction. Its presence in the tissue causes mechanical

irritation which, in turn, encapsulates the foreign body. The reaction is only exudative and fibroplastic in type.

2. Other nonorganized material may interact with the tissue of the eye in chemical reaction which finally produces specific or nonspecific damage.

3. Organized material sets up a proliferative reaction with formation of granulation tissue and giant cells.

The injury caused by a foreign body is determined also by the momentum with which it enters the eye. A large foreign body travelling with sufficient velocity disrupts the whole globe. A small particle with sufficient velocity enters the globe but the main structure of the globe is preserved.

From the clinical point of view, the most important characteristic of a foreign body is its magnetic properties. If a foreign body has a high content of iron, it is magnetic and its removal is relatively easier than that of a nonmagnetic foreign body. The incidence of intraocular magnetic foreign body in industrial accidents is relatively high and, therefore, the percentage of successful removal of intraocular foreign bodies is also high.

Various techniques are available to determine the presence, consistency, and location of an intraocular foreign body. They are as follows:

1. Ophthalmoscopy
2. Slit lamp
3. X-ray (CAT scan)
4. Magnet
5. Metal detector
6. Ultrasound

Direct visualization by slit lamp and ophthalmoscopy (particularly indirect ophthalmoscopy) are the means best suited to detect the presence of an intraocular foreign body (Figs. 6-7A and B). Unfortunately, however, the media of the injured eye may not be clear enough to allow careful examination and to determine the presence or absence of a foreign body. Perforation of the lens capsule can lead to rapid cataract development, thus making impossible proper examination of the posterior segment. Therefore, the first examiner may be the only examiner.

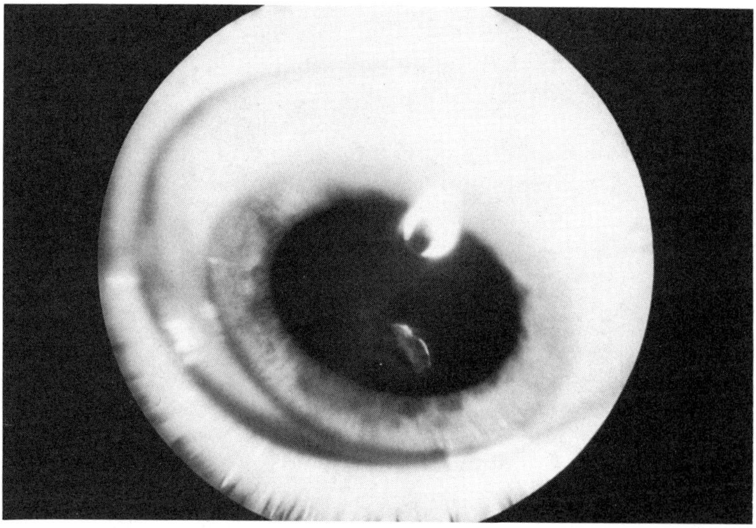

Fig. 6-7A. Metal foreign body in the anterior chamber.

Direct visualization of the anterior chamber with the slit lamp and the gonioprism is sometimes useful to discover an intraocular foreign body in the anterior chamber or in the chamber angle. A transparent foreign body such as glass may be discovered only after careful slit-lamp examination.

In addition to the previously mentioned examination methods, bone-free radiologic techniques should be used in all cases of suspected intraocular foreign body regardless of whether or not a foreign body is detectable with direct observation. In the case of a perforating injury, multiple foreign bodies often may be retained. Occasionally, not all intraocular particles can be seen by direct visualization, and an x-ray examination will detect most of them. CAT scans should be used when necessary (Fig. 6-8).

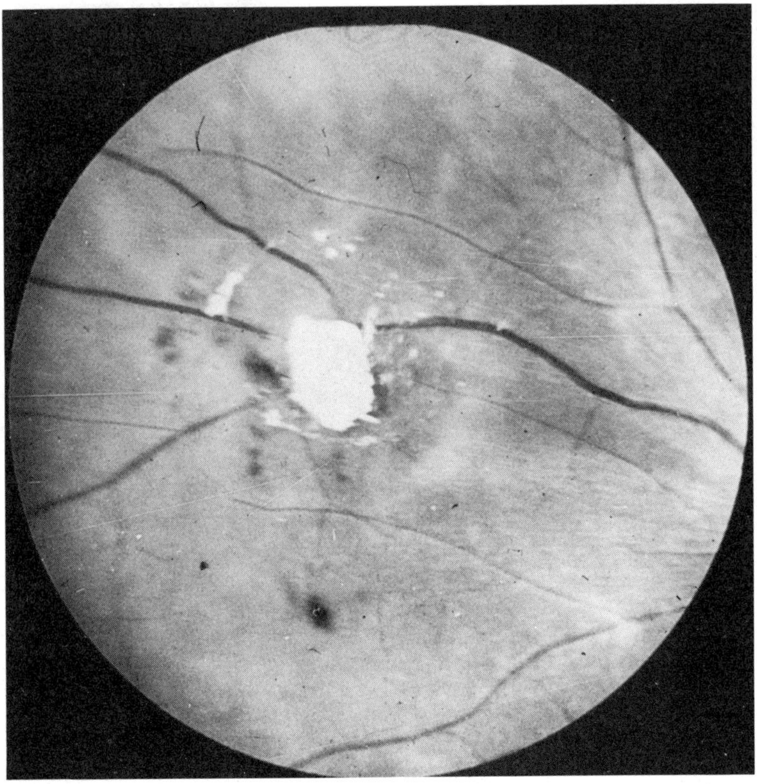

Fig. 6-7B. Intraocular foreign body adherent to the retina.

Radiology may be helpful also in determining the nature of the foreign body. For example, different metals show different shadows on x-ray films. Iron shows a stronger shadow than does aluminum; therefore, by performing an x-ray examination of the globe, one may learn about the chemical constitution of the foreign body. Only an experienced radiologist can make such a determination.

Recently the use of the CAT scan has become very efficacious in evaluating foreign body injuries. The CAT scan is more easily administered in instances such as a severely disrupted globe.

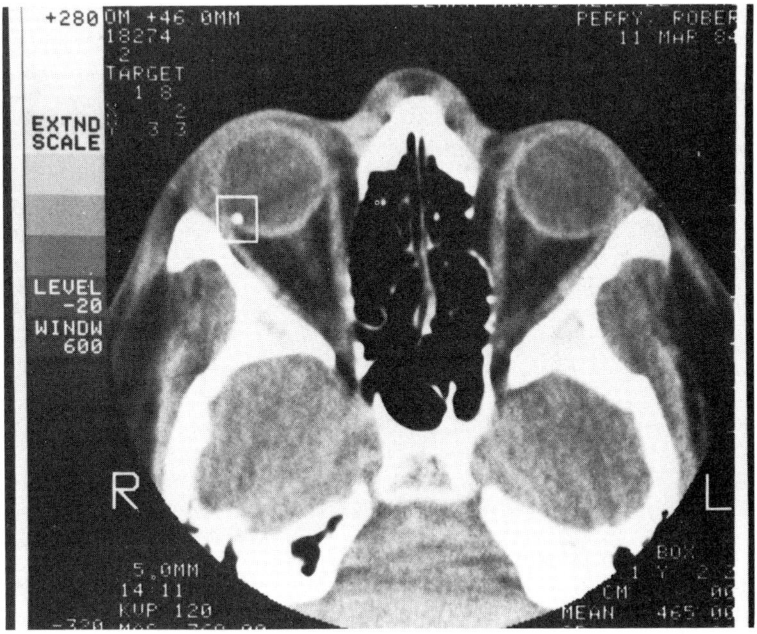

Fig. 6-8. Axial CAT scan showing a foreign body embedded in the retina temporal to the optic disc.

Ultrasonography is one of the newer types of instrumentation used to search for foreign bodies. It may help considerably in the diagnosis and prognosis of eye injuries with or without retained intraocular foreign body.

Guidelines for Treatment

Once the presence and the location of an intraocular foreign body are established, the decision to treat the case surgically or conservatively must be made. In most cases of intraocular foreign body, the prognosis is guarded. Two important goals of the treatment must always be considered: preservation of the eyeball and restoration of useful vision.

Enucleation or evisceration immediately after injury is rarely necessary. In most cases, recovery and restoration of vision is unpredictable at the time of injury. The persistence of light perception is a strong indication to make every effort to remove the foreign body and to preserve the globe. On the other hand, if there is no light perception and disorganization of internal ocular tissues, including the retina and vitreous, then enucleation may be indicated.

It is absolutely necessary that the eye and the entire orbit on the injured side by handled carefully prior to surgical intervention. Occasionally, the eyeball must be closed temporarily before performing the procedures necessary to locate the intraocular foreign body. This is necessary in order to prevent the prolapse of intraocular tissue during radiologic or ultrasonic examination of the globe.

Injured intraocular tissue, in particular, uveal tissue, tends to bleed. Therefore, during diagnostic procedures such as physical examination or x-ray examination, the tissue must be handled gently to prevent secondary bleeding.

As mentioned previously, the reaction of the eye to a foreign body depends largely on the chemical nature of the foreign body and its position within the eye. The physician must be aware of the risk involved in leaving a relatively inert foreign body in the eye and to compare this risk to the surgical risk involved in its removal; finally, he must decide what type of treatment, surgical or conservative, promises better visual acuity. In general, it is hazardous to leave in the eye a foreign body which contains iron or copper. Within a few days copper can cause severe intraocular inflammation which may destroy the eye. A retained foreign body of iron or of copper also may cause late occurring syndromes such as siderosis or chalcosis, respectively. Therefore, early removal of a foreign body of iron or copper is strongly recommended.

On the other hand, a small piece of stone lying on the lower portion of the retina may cause very little disturbance to the vision and very little inflammatory reaction in the eye. In the long range, the stone will be encapsulated by fibrous tissue with very little possibility of late complications or inflammation. Therefore, considering the surgical trauma involved in removing the stone and the complications occurring from an inert intraocular foreign body, it is almost always advisable to leave the intraocular particle untouched. To summarize, the risks involved in leaving a foreign body in the eye must be weighed against the danger of removing it surgically.

The location of the foreign particle in the eye is also of considerable importance in the final decision as to how to treat the injured eye. For example, a foreign object visible in the anterior segment usually is not difficult to remove. The surgical trauma is minimal and, therefore, the decision between surgery and conservative treatment is easily reached. On the other hand, it is more difficult to reach a decision when the same particle is in the vitreous.

The decision to remove the foreign body should be made before the particle becomes encapsulated by fibrous tissue. The encapsulation of the foreign body takes a few days rather than a few hours. This gives the physician enough time to perform the necessary diagnostic tests. Therefore, there is no necessity for the immediate removal of the particle; the decision and the treatment should be carefully planned and executed within a few days after the occurrence of the injury.

LATE COMPLICATIONS OF PERFORATING INJURIES AND PROGNOSIS OF INTRAOCULAR FOREIGN BODIES

SIDEROSIS

Siderosis is a late complication of an intraocular foreign body containing iron. This is a delayed chemical reaction of the ocular tissues to the metallic particle. It is a chronic degenerative process which may result in blindness. The seriousness of the disease depends on the ferrous content of the foreign particle. The less the ferrous content, the less the tendency to siderosis. The exact chemistry of siderosis is not yet understood. It is believed that iron molecules enter the cells. Once within the cells, the iron combines with protein to form an insoluble protein-iron complex which is responsible for the death of the affected cells. It has been observed that certain cells have a special affinity to absorb more iron molecules than others. The most dense deposit of the metal occurs on the anterior surface and the musculature of the iris, the trabecular meshwork of the anterior chamber, the subcapsular epithelium of the lens, the epithelium of the ciliary body, and the peripheral retina.

Siderosis occurs from 2 months to 2 years after injury. Diminution of vision, increased dark adaptation time, night blindness, and concentric contraction of the visual field are definite signs of the disease. Electroretinography (ERG) may help considerably in the early diagnosis of the disease and the prognosis of an eye containing an iron particle. It is believed that removal of the foreign particle in a late stage rarely helps to stop progression of siderosis. However, serial ERGs are important in following the prognosis of intraocular iron content foreign bodies. In later stages of the disease, the deterioration of visual acuity and other signs of the disease are graver and, finally, complete amaurosis develops.

CHALCOSIS

Chalcosis, a disease similar to siderosis, is induced by copper molecules. The preferential deposit of copper is either in or on the limiting membranes of the eye rather than intracellular, as in the case of siderosis. The clinical appearance of the disease is less dramatic and the prognosis is not nearly as poor. Sometimes an eye can retain a copper-containing foreign body for long periods of time without significant loss of vision.

The clinical appearance of chalcosis is characterized by (1) a greenish-blue ring in the peripheral cornea located in Descemet's membrane, (2) a sunflower cataract in the anterior capsule of the lens, (3) impregnation of the zonular fibers, (4) metallic particles in the aqueous humor, (5) greenish coloration of the iris, and (6) copper particles deposited in the vitreous and on the surface of the retina. A similar clinical picture can be observed in Wilson's disease (hepatolenticular degeneration) which is actually an endogenous chalcosis.

Specific treatment for chalcosis is still not available and ultimate visual loss is likely from a retained foreign body containing copper.

SYMPATHETIC OPHTHALMITIS

Sympathetic ophthalmitis is a rare disease which may occur after a perforating injury of the eye, particularly if the uveal tissue is injured or prolapses and remains so for some time. The disease is a bilateral, granulomatous uveitis originating in the injured eye. The onset of inflammation in the fellow (uninjured) eye is usually within 3 weeks to 2 months after injury; however, inflammation in the fellow eye occurring from 9 days to many years after ocular trauma has been reported. In untreated cases of iris or ciliary body prolapse, sympathetic ophthalmitis may occur in as high as 5% of cases. The incidence of this disease in modern ophthalmology, however, has diminished greatly. Prompt and precise posttraumatic surgery, early enucleation if necessary, and the introduction of corticosteroid therapy account for the marked decline in the incidence of sympathetic ophthalmitis.

Corticosteroids given topically, subconjunctivally, and systemically after injury may prevent the development of the disease. Once the noninjured eye shows signs of granulomatous uveitis, it is doubtful whether enucleation of the injured eye is beneficial to prevent further progression of the disease. Untreated cases tend to be progressive and about 50% lose useful vision.

TRAUMATIC CYSTS

The development of cysts within the eye after a perforating injury is an uncommon complication. An organized foreign body retained within the eye may result in cyst formation. An epithelial implantation cyst may follow a perforating injury. In the cornea, epithelial cells grow into the wound or small fragments of the epithelium are detached and transplanted to another layer. Epithelial proliferation may form a cyst in the anterior chamber. Sometimes several cysts may coexist at the same time. Implantation cysts within the globe are relatively rare. The diagnosis of these intraocular cysts is not important at the time of initial injury as they occur weeks to months later. Secondary glaucoma may develop in an eye with an implantation cyst. The history of perforating injury is always an important factor in making the correct diagnosis. The treatment of these intraocular cysts is usually surgical. While the surgical removal of cysts is sometimes successful, ultimate consequences of cysts are usually serious.

BIBLIOGRAPHY

Brinton, G.S. et al.: Posterior segment trauma. Amer J Ophthal 93(3):271-8, 1982.

Cinotti, A.A. and Maltzman, B.A.: Prognosis and treatment of perforating ocular injuries. Ophthal Surg 6(4):54, 1975.

Coleman, D.J.: Early vitrectomy for severe ocular trauma. Amer J Ophthal 93(5):543-51, 1982.

Consumer Products Guide -- U.S. Consumer Product Safety Commission Report. U.S. Government Printing Office, Washington, D.C. (Oct) 1974.

Duke-Elder, S.: System of Ophthalmology, Injuries. Vol. XIV. Henry Kimpton, London, and Mosby, St. Louis, 1972.

Forster, R.K. et al.: Management of infectious endophthalmitis. Ophthal 87(4):313-9, 1980.

Freeman, M.H. (ed.): Ocular Trauma. Appleton-Century-Crofts, NY, 1979.

Gombos, G.M.: Ocular war injuries in Jerusalem during the 1967 Arab-Israeli conflict. Amer J Ophthal 68:474, 1969.

Hoefle, F.B.: Initial treatment of eye injuries. Arch Ophthal 79:33, 1968.

Karpe, G.: Early diagnosis of siderosis retinae by the use of electroretinography. Docum Ophthal 2:227, 1948.

Lim, J.K.S. and Cinotti, A.A.: Review of 890 consecutive enucleations. Annals of Ophthal 8(7):865-69, 1976.

Machemer, R., Posel, J.M. and Buettner, H.: A new concept for vitreous surgery -- 1. Instrumentation. Am J Ophthal 73:1, 1972.

Machemer, R.: A new concept for vitreous surgery -- 2. Surgical technique and complications. Am J Ophthal 74:1022, 1972.

Mackensen, G. and Fauborn, F.: Primary and secondary reconstruction of the eyeball after extensive lacerations. Ophth Surg 5:43, 1974.

Macrae, W.E. and Macrae, H.M.: Serious eye injuries caused by intraocular foreign bodies. Need they be disabling? Can J Ophthal 1:291, 1972.

Maltzman, B.A., Eng, K. and Cinotti, A.A.: Perforating Ocular Injuries – A Second Look. J Med Soc NJ 75(4):317, 1978.

Michels, R.G.: Vitrectomy methods in penetrating ocular trauma. Ophthal 87(7):62-45, 1980.

Paton, D. and Goldberg, M.F.: Management of Ocular Injuries. Saunders, Philadelphia, 1976.

Roper-Hall, M. J.: Perforating ocular injuries. Proceedings of the Royal Society of Medicine 60:597, 1967.

Slusher, M. M. et al.: Management of intraretinal foreign bodies. Ophthal 89(4):369-73, 1982.

Symposium of the New Orleans Academy of Ophthalmology. Industrial and Traumatic Ophthalmology. Mosby, St. Louis, 1964.

Troutman, R. C. (ed.): Microsurgery of Ocular Injuries. Third Int Symp Ophthal Microsurg Study Group, Merida, Yucatan, Mexico, 1970. Adv Ophth, Karger, Basel, 1972.

Troutman, R. C.: Operating microscope in ophthalmic surgery. Trans Am Ophth Soc 63:335, 1965.

Zagora, E.: Eye Injuries. Charles C Thomas, Springfield, 1970.

Chapter 7

TRAUMA TO THE OPTIC NERVE

CONCUSSION INJURY OF THE OPTIC NERVE

The optic nerve of each eye is composed of more than one million axons which arise from ganglion cells of the retina. The optic nerve is approximately 50 mm in length. It may be divided into four components: an intraocular portion measuring approximately 1 mm, an orbital portion behind the globe measuring approximately 30 mm, an intracanalicular portion measuring approximately 6 mm, and an intracranial portion measuring approximately 10 mm.

Injury to the optic nerve is relatively common in concussion injuries. The optic nerve may be injured as a result of frontal or frontotemporal injury. There may be soft tissue ecchymosis around the eye and proptosis from hemorrhage and edema within the orbit. Any patient with severe proptosis should be evaluated by an ophthalmologist on an emergency basis because of the possibility of compression of the optic nerve circulation. In all cases, standard radiologic views of the orbit should be ordered to rule out a concomitant orbital fracture. Actual involvement of the bony optic canal is found only in a minority of cases and is best established by optic canal tomography and CT scan.

A bony spicule within the optic foramen may cause compression of the optic nerve and account for immediate loss of vision after the injury. The immediate loss of vision after injury suggests one of two mechanisms: either an actual tear in the optic nerve or a concussive injury that interrupts the blood supply. Hemorrhages or edema in the canal may cause such an obstruction. Patients may have an altitudinal hemianopsia that is usually inferior from a concussive injury to the optic nerve within the optic canal.

With concussive injury to the optic nerve, the only abnormality on ophthalmoscopy may be optic nerve hemorrhages. In general, vision starts to return within a few days and reaches a maximum return in 3 or 4 weeks. Optic disc pallor will begin in 2-3 weeks after the injury. Because of the possibilities of secondary edema causing compression of the blood supply to the optic nerve, the administration of systemic steroids may be helpful in reducing the compressive effects from the edema and help in restoring vision. If the loss of vision occurred at the moment of the trauma, it is unlikely that recovery of vision would be enhanced by therapy. If it can be established, however, that there had been vision, even if for only a few moments, the loss of vision may be recoverable. In such cases, emergency intervention such as surgical removal of the roof of the optic canal may be beneficial, although this surgery is controversial.

As would be expected in an optic nerve lesion, pupillary size would be unchanged, but a Marcus Gunn pupillary response would be found. Consensual reactions in the emergency room will help to distinguish between an optic nerve and oculomotor nerve injury as a cause of the nonreacting pupil. In a third nerve palsy, the eyeball is usually in a downward and outward position and the pupil may be dilated. Traumatic avulsions of the optic nerve may sever the central retinal artery; and on ophthalmoscopy, perfusion of the retinal vessels will not be seen. The optic nerve, however, will take several weeks to develop pallor.

Related head injuries including subdural and subarachnoid hemorrhages may result in retinal hemorrhages. The syndrome in which increased intracranial pressure causes optic nerve, retinal, and vitreal hemorrhages is known as Terson's syndrome.

An injury to the optic chiasm may occur when the fracture that crosses the region of the sella turcica and the optic chiasm also may be torn by severe injuries. A pure chiasmal injury produces a bitemporal hemianopsia. But, more commonly, the chiasmal injury is combined with a more obvious optic nerve injury on one side.

In general, the differential diagnosis of loss of vision following trauma includes:

- Direct trauma to the optic nerve
- The pressure of lid swelling causing compression of the optic nerve
- Vitreal hemorrhage
- Blood or foreign material within the eye
- Traumatic cataract and/or luxation of the lens
- Central artery or vein occlusion
- Traumatic retinal edema and hemorrhage
- Retinal detachment
- Episode of acute angle-closure glaucoma
- Hysteria
- Malingering

RUPTURE AND EVULSION OF THE OPTIC NERVE

The most common cause of a rupture and avulsion of the optic nerve is a penetrating injury involving the eye and orbit. It may also result from severe direct concussion to the globe. Very often such an injury is associated with intraocular hemorrhage. The rupture of the nerve may be complete or partial. In general, the ophthalmologic appearance of a complete rupture reveals partial or complete absence of the vessels. The vision is gravely impaired and the visual loss is irreversible. Unfortunately, there is no effective treatment.

BIBLIOGRAPHY

Cogan, D. G.: Neurology of the Visual System. Charles C. Thomas, Springfield, Ill., 1966.

Duke-Elder, S.: System of Ophthalmology. Injuries. Vol. XIV. Mosby, St. Louis, 1972.

Walsh, F. B.: Pathological-clinical correlations. 1. Indirect trauma to the optic nerves and chiasm. Invest Ophthal 5:433, 1966.

Walsh, F. B. and Hoyt, W. F.: Clinical Neuro-Ophthalmology, 3rd ed. Williams and Wilkins, Baltimore, 1969.

Chapter 8

TRAUMA OF THE EYELIDS, ORBIT, AND ADNEXA

Injury to the eyelids and orbit may be part of multiple trauma to the body. Stabilization of vital bodily functions takes precedence over primary repair of injured lid tissues. At times, repair of lid structures may be planned at the same time as the repair of more vital structures of the body. Because of the great vascularity of the eyelids, primary repair can be delayed days and even weeks. Before repair of lid and orbital tissues is undertaken, a history, physical examination, and appropriate x-ray studies must be performed. Any injury involving the lids and orbits should be evaluated by an ophthalmologist to rule out ocular involvement. Calling an ophthalmologist several days after an injury may lead to a serious medicolegal problem. At times, a multidisciplinary approach is necessary for the treatment of head and facial injuries. Ear, nose, and throat surgeons, general plastic surgeons, neurosurgeons, and ophthalmologic surgeons are sometimes required for the evaluation and treatment of patients. This chapter will first consider the eyelid injuries. It will later evaluate orbital anatomy and injuries.

TYPES OF EYELID INJURIES

LACERATING INJURIES

These injuries are commonly caused by sharp edges of glass or metal. They are frequently encountered in automobile accidents. No loss of tissue is expected. The edges of the wound usually lie in good apposition, with edema occasionally causing some slight displacement. Adjacent to the lacerated areas may be heavily abraded skin surfaces ingrained with dirt or grease. These areas must be thoroughly scrubbed to prevent a tatooing which requires dermabrasion months after complete healing has taken place. The foreign body may be irrigated from the wound during preparation for surgery or may be palpated and removed. Penetrating wounds may show only a small wound of entry but must be carefully explored. The intracranial tissues may be involved with major central nervous complication. Umbrella tips, automobile aerials, and sharp sticks are common offenders.

Puncture wounds of the lids caused by sharp-tipped objects, especially metal-tipped darts, may conceal a perforating injury of the globe. Even if the site of lid puncture seems remote, visual acuity and careful indirect ophthalmoscopy may reveal a perforating injury of the globe.

DISRUPTION AND PARTIAL AVULSION

When a direct blow to the eye is sufficiently violent to avulse the lid, ruptures of the posterior globe must be considered. The structures of the ruptured lid are irregular but may be easily reconstructed (Fig. 8-1). A glancing blow on the nasal side can partially avulse either or both lids at a point between the medial canthus and the puncta. All medially located lacerations or avulsions must be carefully inspected to determine the integrity of the lacrimal drainage apparatus. An attempt must always be made to repair the canaliculi since the loss of function to only one canaliculus may affect tear drainage.

Total avulsion of either or both lids is rare but may occur after human and animal bites of the lids. The portion of missing lid may be used in the repair. The survival of at least the tarsal structures may be of great assistance in the reconstruction and avoids the use of substitutes such as nasal or ear cartilage.

Systematic evaluation of the injuries should be carried out as follows:

1. If the state of consciousness allows, measure the visual acuity using a reading card or Snellen chart with eyeglasses if available, or a multiple pinhole. The medicolegal implications cannot be overemphasized.

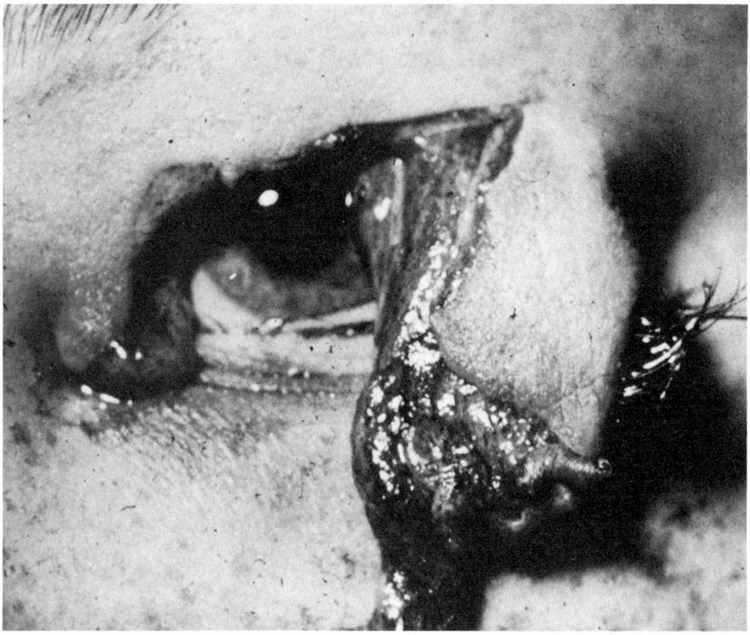

Fig. 8-1. Partial avulsion of lid.

2. Inspect the wounds using intense illumination and determine whether the globe is involved.

3. Irrigate the wound depths freely and, using sterile gloves and pad, determine if the wounds involve bone. Palpate for crepitation. Determine if there has been any involvement of lacrimal structure or levator muscle by the presence of fat gaping through the wound.

4. The presence of a foreign body should always be considered and orbital plain films obtained (see Orbital Section).

5. Administration of tetanus antitoxin or tetanus toxoid must be considered at the time of admission to the hospital or emergency room.

SURGICAL TREATMENT

Small lacerations can be repaired under local anesthesia by local infiltration in the emergency room. Lacerations that involve the canaliculus, levator, or lid margin are usually better repaired in the operating room. Supraorbital, frontal, and infraorbital nerve block may be helpful (Figs. 8-2 and 8-3). The

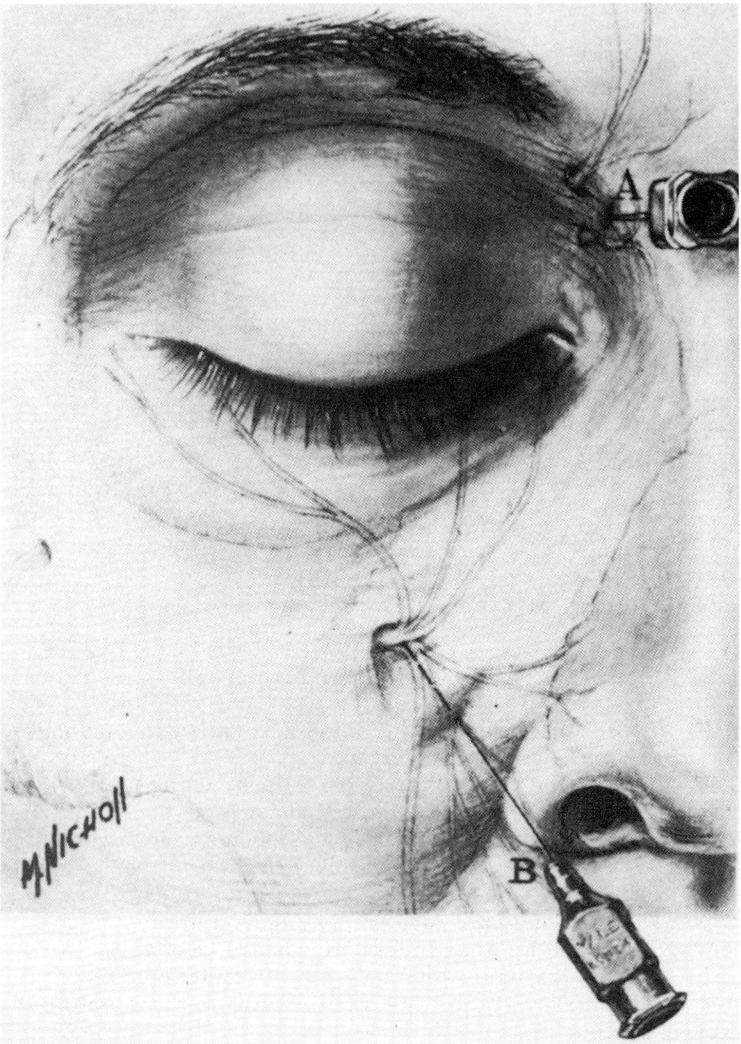

Fig. 8-2. Anesthesia of the (A) supratrochlear and (B) infratrochlear nerves. (Reprinted with the permission of the publisher and the author.) Callahan, A.: Reconstructive surgery of the eyelids and ocular adnexa. Aesculapius Pub. Co., Birmingham.

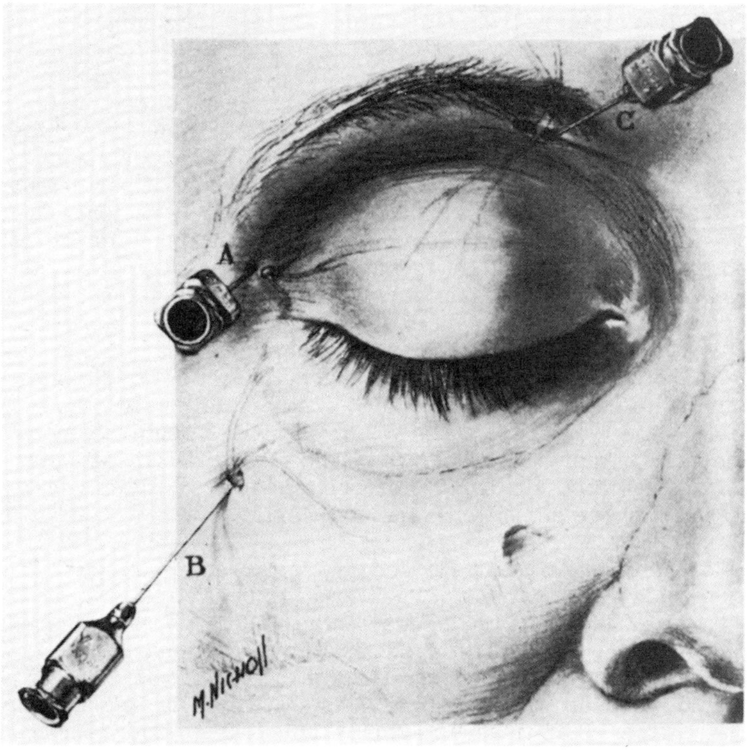

Fig. 8-3. Anesthesia of the (A) lacrimal, (B) zygomaticofacial, (C) supraorbital nerves. (Reprinted with the permission of the publisher and the author.) Callahan, A.: Reconstructive surgery of the eyelids and ocular adnexa. Aesculapius Pub. Co., Birmingham.

frontal nerve divides into the supratrochlear and supraorbital branches approximately 4 cm behind the superior orbital rim. Because this area has no major blood vessels, a 4-cm-long needle, usually 25 gauge, may be passed at the middle of the superior orbital rim. The needle must not penetrate the levator muscle and, therefore, must creep along the roof of the orbit for approximately 4 cm. Penetration of the periosteum will result in ineffective anesthesia. The block is purely sensory and, theoretically, should not affect the levator muscle activity. The risk of retrobulbar hemorrhage is small yet possible. For this reason, this block should not be utilized if there is any possibility of a ruptured globe.

The infraorbital nerve supplies the skin and the conjunctiva of the lower lid. The infraorbital foramen contains the infraorbital nerve, its artery, and vein, and is located approximately one thumb-width lateral to the ala of the nose and one thumb superior. One and one-half to two cc's of local anesthetic using a short (one-half inch) needle is useful. A finger placed at the orbital rim is helpful in preventing inadvertent perforation of the globe or the orbital tissues. In addition to regional anesthesia, facial muscle akinesia may be accomplished to prevent lid squeezing. A Van Lint technique is usually adequate. The Van Lint technique utilizes local infiltration of the anesthetic into the deep subcutaneous tissues along the orbital margins and in the lateral canthal area. In general, 300 mg of lidocaine (30 ml of 1% lidocaine without epinephrine) (50 ml of 1% lidocaine with epinephrine 1/100,000) can be safely used. Ruptured globes, in association with lid injuries, require general anesthesia to prevent pressure on the globe by infiltration of local anesthetic. Removal of an orbital foreign body is generally performed under general anesthesia.

Betadine as preparation for surgery is extremely effective. In its diluted form, it has not been found to be irritating to the eye. After anesthesia has been administered, repeated inspection of the wound is carried out. A microscope may be required to identify the severed ends of the canaliculi. Time should be spent arranging the jigsaw puzzle of lid lacerations. The vitality of lid tissues is remarkable and it is not necessary that tissue be removed.

SIMPLE LACERATIONS OF THE LID WITHOUT LOSS OF TISSUE

All wounds should be debrided and foreign bodies removed. Copious irrigation of the wound with antibiotic solutions is important. When examining a lid laceration, damage to the levator, canaliculi, and lacrimal gland should always be ruled out. Prolapse of fat through a lid wound indicates that the orbital septum has been violated and that the levator should be examined when the lid is explored in the operating room. Traumatic dehiscenses of the levator from its insertion at the level of the upper tarsal border should be repaired. Lacerations of the orbital septum are best left unsutured because of the late scarring and consequent shortening of the septum resulting in lagophthalmos. Severe or complete ptosis after trauma may be secondary to a levator muscle hematoma or nerve injury and may improve with time. If no wound is present, and traumatic ptosis is present, the patient should be observed. Spontaneous correction of traumatic ptosis may occur over a year or longer.

Medial Canthal Tendon Lacerations

The medial canthal tendon is an extension of tarsus that has a superior and inferior crus that combine to form a common tendon. Lacerations of a medial canthal tendon will present with telecanthus. In addition, lacrimal sac damage should be anticipated. If only one crus of the medial canthal tendon, that is, the inferior crus, is injured, a canalicular laceration is usually also present. Blunting of the lateral canthal angle suggests lateral canthal tendon damage. Attention to the anatomic insertion of the medial and lateral canthal tendons is warranted for restoration of lid function and cosmesis. Nonabsorbable sutures that include bites into the deep soft tissue may be adequate. In more severe injuries, transnasal wiring of the medial canthal tendon or wiring of the lateral canthus to the inside of the lateral orbital rim is probably best performed as a secondary nonemergency repaired when tissue edema subsides (Figs. 8-4A and B).

Simple skin muscle lacerations that do not involve the septum or underlying levator require suturing of skin edges only (Fig. 8-5). The orbicularis muscle layer is not sutured separately. When suturing skin and muscle lacerations in the medial canthal area, as in canalicular lacerations, it is important to recognize that the temporal edge of a vertical or oblique laceration will contract towards the lateral canthal tendon and down towards the cheek from gravity. When suturing the skin edges, the bites in the temporal edge of the wound must be more superior than the bites in the nasal edge of the wound to compensate for this tendency.

Identification of Eyelid Landmarks

Skin landmarks, including brow and lid margins, should first be identified and sutured when repairing a complex lid laceration. Skin defects may be repaired by underlying skin muscle flaps and advancing such flaps. Lacerations of the lid should be aligned by first suturing the upper border of the tarsus and the lid margin (Figs. 8-6 and 8-7). In the lower lid tarsus, two absorbable sutures are sufficient while in the upper lid tarsus, three such sutures are necessary. The vertical dimension of the upper tarsus is 10 mm, while that of the lower tarsus is only 5 mm. This discrepancy accounts for the difference in the number of sutures necessary for apposition of the lacerated tarsus.

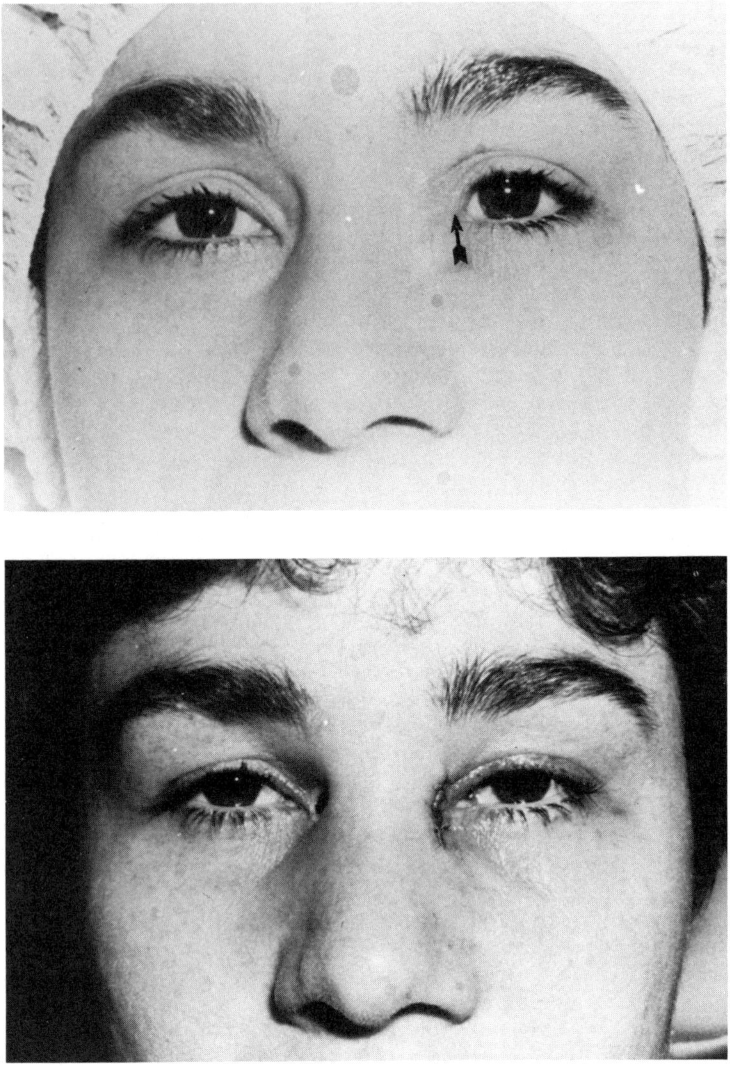

Figs. 8-4A and B. Telecanthus (A) on left side (arrow), from horse hoof trauma repaired by transnasal wiring (B).

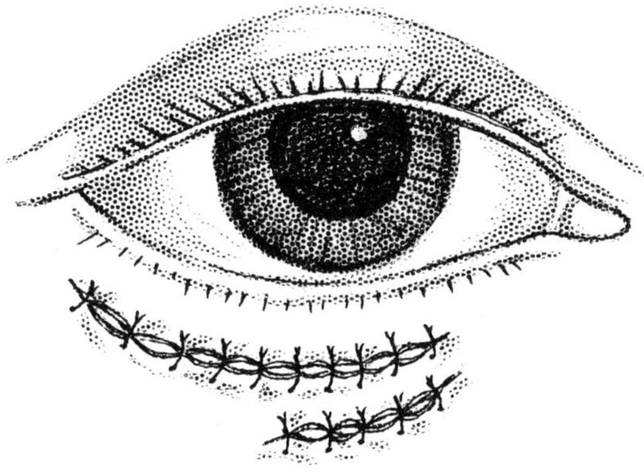

Fig. 8-5. Closure of skin laceration parallel with the orbicularis muscle.

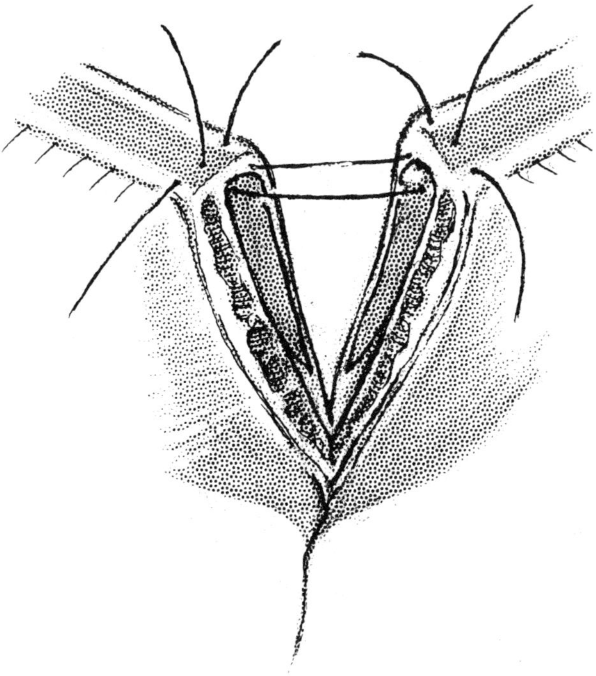

Fig. 8-6. Closure of vertical lacerations; marginal aligning sutures are shown.

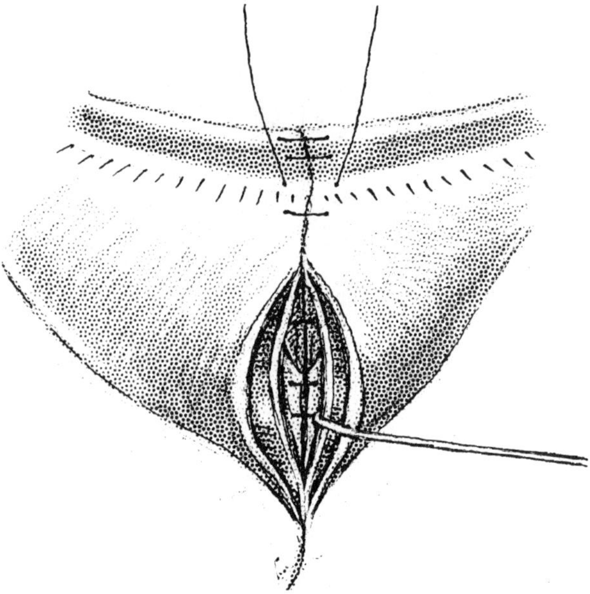

Fig. 8-7. Closure of vertical laceration with interrupted chronic suture.

Lid margin lacerations are sutured using 6-0 sutures (Fig. 8-6). One 6-0 silk suture should be placed at the gray line or just posterior to the gray line at the level of the meibomian orifices. The bites should be of a depth and length of approximately 1-2 mm on each side of the wound, which is 2-3 meibomian orifices. Two additional 6-0 silk sutures should be placed, one just anterior and one just posterior to the central suture. The centrally placed suture may be a 5-0 suture for stability. The anterior and posterior sutures have bites that are slightly shorter and less deep than the central suture. All lid margin sutures are incorporated into one of the skin sutures that is used to appose the vertical laceration. In this way, the cornea is not abraded. These lid margin sutures are incorporated after two throws, so that the skin does not undergo pressure necrosis by the lid margin sutures, which would otherwise lie directly on the skin. The conjunctiva need not be sutured. A 4-0 silk transmarginal traction suture that enters and exits through the gray line in one bite may be used to immobilize the lid to prevent contractures of the vertically oriented

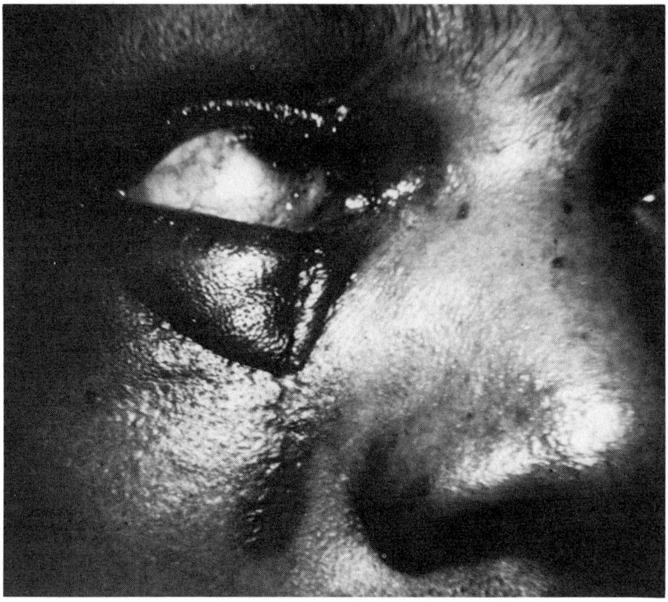

Fig. 8-8. Vertical laceration causing notching and retraction of the lower lid.

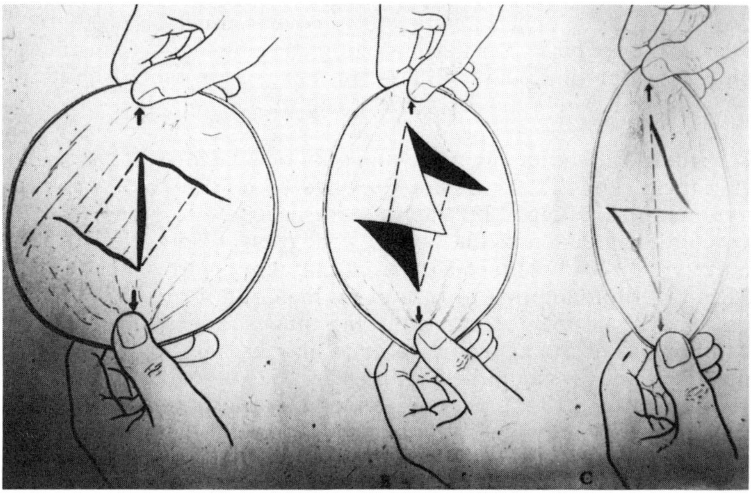

Fig. 8-9. The principle of Z-plasty.

lacerations. Z-plasties are rarely necessary to prevent lid notching, unless there is loss of tissue (Figs. 8-8 and 8-9). The traction suture may be taped to the brow with slight traction in the case of the lower lid laceration or to the cheek in the case of the upper lid laceration. Alternatively, the upper and lower lids may be sutured together by using a horizontal mattress type suture that starts approximately 3 mm from the lid margin through the skin on each side that goes through the gray line. These sutures are tied over a cotton pledget to prevent pressure necrosis of the skin by the suture.

LID LACERATIONS WITH LOSS OF TISSUE

These injuries are best repaired in the operating room. Primary union of a lid laceration is possible if one-fourth or less of the lid margin is lost. By performing a canthotomy and cantholysis of the superior or inferior crus of the lateral canthal tendon, larger defects may be repaired. Up to 50% of an upper lid or lower lid defect may be closed by a semicircular flap of Tenzel. Larger lower lid defects may be closed by a Hughes tarsoconjunctival flap. Similar large defects of the upper lid may be closed by a Cutler-Beard technique. Both of these procedures are described elsewhere in detail. Edematous necrotic tissues are probably best repaired at a later date, because the tissues will not tolerate further surgical trauma and will break apart if stress is placed on them. In addition, large noncosmetic scars will result. Ice compresses and antibiotics are utilized until the edema subsides. The cornea must be protected during this period. Ophthalmologic consultation is important. Ointments or ointments with saran wrap or protective plastic shields or bubbles are extremely useful.

Irregular ragged or necrotic margins of lacerations should be trimmed. Loss of tissue must always be minimized. A vertical avulsion of the upper lid that results in loss of only part of the vertical dimension of the tarsus will cause a lid notch, if primarily repaired without removing the remainder of the tarsus. This principle applies to loss of tissues either at the lid margin or at the superior border of the tarsus. A canthotomy with cantholysis of the appropriate crus may be necessary. All lid margin wounds should be repaired in a pentagontal fashion rather than a "V" fashion. This technique insures equal distribution of tension on both sides of the laceration and prevents lid notching.

General Principles Regarding Lid Reconstruction

In general, the lid must contain a skin layer and a mucosal layer in order to maintain integrity of globe. Where there is a loss of tissue, an advancement flap of skin and a tarsal conjunctival flap from the apposing lid may be utilized to reconstruct the anterior and posterior lamellae, respectively. In either case, the normal lid margin should not be violated. Occasional skin grafts or mucous membrane grafts from the mucosa of the lower lip or from the buccal mucosa are necessary. A graft may be placed over a flap, but lack of blood supply will result in failure when a graft is placed over a graft. The use of a Z-plasty may be helpful in obtaining additional skin tissue. Excision of resultant (burrows) triangles is usually necessary.

REPAIR OF CANALICULAR INJURIES

The integrity of the lacrimal system is necessary for its proper function. Any lid lacerations nasal to the punctum should be considered to involve the canaliculus, and the patient should be evaluated by an ophthalmologist. Repair of lacerations of the canaliculus is best done by an ophthalmologist or ophthalmic plastic surgeon under general anesthesia using the operating microscope. The use of the Worst pigtail probe is discouraged because of the necessity to pass the probe blindly through the delicate common internal punctum into the area of the lacerated canaliculus (Fig. 8-10). Instead, a technique using a stent through the severed canaliculus alone is favored (Fig. 8-11). A wire stent can be used for one or both canaliculi simultaneously.

Injuries that lead to loss of large amounts of a canaliculus or lacrimal sac are probably secondarily repaired at a later date with a Jones tube by an ophthalmic plastic surgeon.

BURNS OF THE EYELIDS

The types of burns that involve the eyelids include chemical burns, both acid and alkali, and thermal burns. Alkali burns are more severe than acid burns of the lids. The same general principles that apply to the treatment of chemical burns pertain to thermal burns of the lid. The main problem with the eyelid is the development of cicatricial ectropion and exposure keratitis. In general, any surgical repair of the lids may be delayed for 3-4 weeks. The time honored treatment has been a temporary or permanent one or two pillar tarsorrhaphy that

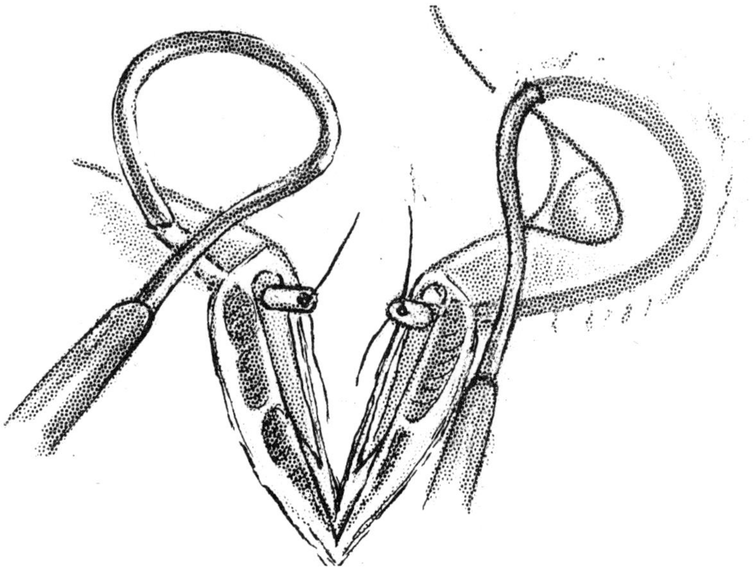

Fig. 8-10. Pigtail probes introduced into canaliculus must traverse normal common internal punctum.

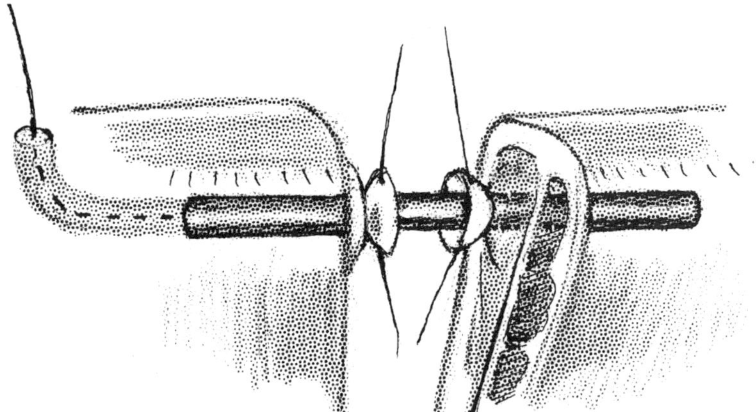

Fig. 8-11. Canalicular stent in place.

acts as a splint to prevent contracture of the lid structures and a twisted, distorted tarsal plate. Others have favored early skin grafting over tarsorrhaphy because they believe that the tarsorrhaphy does not prevent distortion of the lid structure.

The acute problem necessitates the use of antibacterial sulfadiene creams to prevent infections, daily cleansing of the wounds with soap and irrigation with peroxide. Daily debridement is also important. The cornea must be kept moist.

ORBITAL TRAUMA

SURGICAL ANATOMY OF THE ORBIT

The bony orbit is a four-walled (superior, inferior, medial, and lateral) pyramidal structure whose main function is to support and protect the eye. The superior and lateral margins are particularly strong and shield the globe from direct trauma. The medial and inferior rims of the orbit are less strong, yet their thin walls are designed to fracture or "blow-out" and thus protect the globe from blunt, nonpenetrating trauma.

An understanding of the surgical anatomy of the orbit is helpful in evaluating patients with orbital trauma. The roof of the orbit is composed anteriorly by the frontal bone and posteriorly by the lesser wing of the sphenoid bone. The supraorbital nerve and vessels course in the supraorbital notch in the medial one-third of the orbital roof at its rim. The trochlea of the superior oblique muscle is located at the most medial aspect of the roof. The medial wall contains the lacrimal fossa. The anterior ethmoidal vessels and nerve are located 2. 5 cm behind the orbital rim at the level of the cribiform plate. The orbital floor contains the infraorbital nerve and vessels in the infraorbital groove. These structures exit through the infraorbital foramen.

RADIOLOGICAL VIEWS OF THE ORBIT

The standard radiological views of the orbit include: (a) Caldwell (modified posterior-anterior), (b) Water's, (c) optic canal, (d) lateral, (e) base (submentovertex), (f) tomography and steroscopy, if indicated, and (g) CT scan with coronal and axial views, if performed. The Water's view is optimal for orbital floor fractures, while the basal view shows zygomatic fractures. The lateral orbital view is best for visualization of foreign bodies. Orbital CT scan, particularly the coronal views, often demonstrates the relationship of the orbital soft tissues to the fracture more clearly than plain films or tomography. Multiple orbital and facial fractures may be better demonstrated by tomograms rather than by CT scan. Patients with enophthalmos are best evaluated by tomograms that demonstrate the extent of the orbital floor fracture. Large defects may respond to surgical intervention and placement of an orbital floor implant.

ORBITAL FRACTURES

In this age of high-acceleration motorcycle and automobile accidents and violent traumatic crimes, the variety of possible orbit and facial fractures is limitless. However, certain fractures occur with sufficient regularity that allow classification of orbital fractures into five basic types: (1) floor fractures, (2) medial wall fractures, (3) roof fractures, (4) lateral wall fractures, and (5) combined fractures including tripod, naso-orbital, and LeFort, (types I-III). This classification defines orbital fractures as either internal or external fractures. Internal fractures spare the orbital rim, while external fractures involve the rim.

Orbital Floor (Blow-Out) Fractures

Blow-out fractures are the result of a blunt, nonpenetrating injury that causes a sudden increase in intraorbital pressure. The object which produces the trauma is usually larger than the bony orbital entrance. The resultant hydraulic pressure is transmitted throughout the orbit. Since the inferior and medial walls are the thinnest of the orbit, these structures dissipate the increased intraorbital pressure and fracture. In this way, the eyeball is relatively protected from rupture. Because the mechanism of medial wall fractures is the same as that of a blow-out fracture involving the floor, a medial wall fracture can be considered a form of blow-out fracture. In one series of twenty orbital floor fractures, eight of the patients had a concomitant medial wall fracture. In none of the cases was an isolated medial wall fracture present.

The clinical signs of orbital floor fracture most commonly include traumatic ptosis, hypesthesia in the distribution of the second division of the fifth cranial nerve, subconjunctival and lid hemorrhage, vertical diplopia due to difficulty in elevation or depression and exophthalmos or enophthalmos. Rarely, the

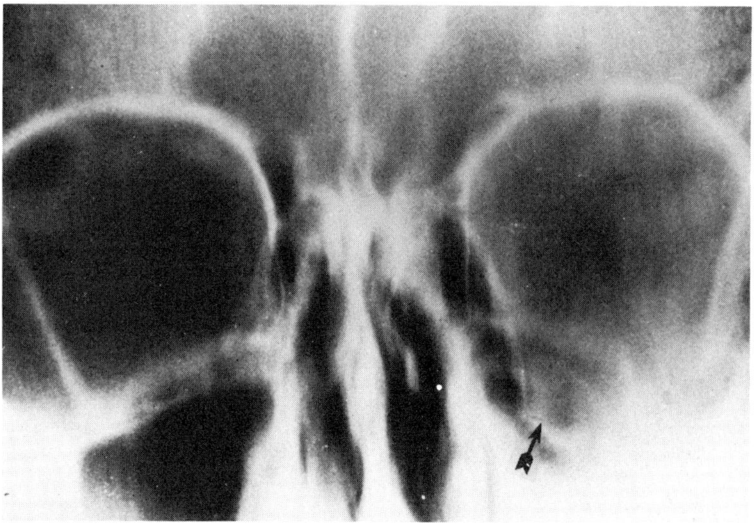

Fig. 8-12. Orbital tomogram shows blow-out fracture present on left side (arrow) with left maxillary clouding.

entire globe prolapses into the maxillary sinus. Initially, extravasated blood may cause exophthalmos and makes evaluation of motility difficult. For this reason, surgery is usually not considered until approximately 1 week after injury. Patients with suspected blow-out fractures in the emergency room should have orbital films taken that day and examination by an ophthalmologist because of possible concomitant eye injuries.

Radiologically, blood may produce an air fluid level in the maxillary sinus. Blood may be present in the sinus without a fracture. A subperiosteal hematoma may be mistaken radiologically for a true floor fracture. Of the standard orbital views the Water's view provides the optimum view of the orbital floor. Tomograms are crucial in difficult cases. (Fig. 8-12). The posterior part of the medial floor is the most common fracture site. The trapdoor variety of blow-out fracture results in entrapment of orbital tissues with positive forced ductions, yet because there is little bony displacement, an orbital floor fracture is difficult to document radiographically. Because of the CT scan's ability to demonstrate soft tissues, CT coronal views may be helpful in such cases (Fig. 8-13).

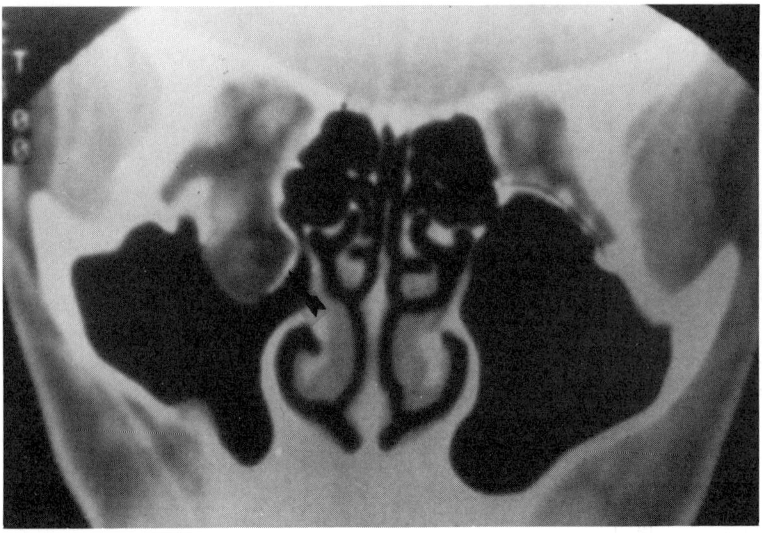

Fig. 8-13. Coronal orbital CT scan shows orbital floor fracture (arrow).

The indications for surgical intervention include diplopia in an important field of gaze, positive forced ductions, and radiological evidence of a floor fracture. If a large floor fracture can be demonstrated usually by orbital tomograms, prevention of late enophthalmos is a possible indication for surgical exploration and insertion of an alloplastic floor implant. These fractures need not be repaired within a few days of injury and optimally are repaired 7-14 days after injury, after edema resolves and before fibrosis begins. Floor defects can be repaired months or even years later. Patients that show improvements in motility are probably better observed. A traumatic ptosis may take 6 months to a year to resolve. Blindness due to compression of the optic nerve circulation is a well known, although rare, complication of orbital floor exploration with or without insertion of an alloplastic implant.

Medial Wall Fracture

The pathophysiology of medial wall fractures caused by a nonpenetrating orbital injury is identical to that of an orbital floor blow-out fracture. Other types of medial wall fractures will be discussed under combined fractures. The signs of a medial wall fracture include orbital emphysema with crepitus under the skin and/or conjunctiva. Crepitus is extremely common in medial wall fractures, and occurs whenever there is a fracture of the common bony wall between the orbit and an adjacent sinus. Epistaxis is often present. As with any orbital floor fracture, significant lid, subconjunctival, and orbital hemorrhage and edema may cause transient exophthalmos. Motility disturbances are rare with medial wall fracture and, if present, may resolve with resorbing blood and decreasing chemosis. As with orbital floor fractures, traumatic muscle palsy due to nerve palsy or intramuscular hemorrhage may simulate entrapment. Difficulty in adduction or abduction with narrowing of the lid fissure in abduction is due to entrapment of the orbital soft tissues adjacent to the medial rectus within the fracture site. Isolated medial wall fractures are extremely rare, and if any vertical motility disturbance is present, an associated orbital floor fracture should be suspected.

Ethmoid fractures are sometimes difficult to identify with standard orbital films because of the overlapping shadows (Figs. 8-14A and B). Ethmoid clouding due to hemorrhage may be the only definite clue. Documenting an ethmoid fracture with tomography is only necessary if there is evidence of entrapment of the medial rectus muscles with a positive forced duction. Some have advocated stereoscopic views. Orbital CT scan with coronal views are extremely helpful. When surgical release of the entrapped tissues is warranted, an incision is made above the lacrimal sac and the periosteum is freed from the underlying bony orbit until the incarcerated tissues are identified.

Penetrating trauma, as opposed to blunt trauma, may result in a medial wall fracture, as well as fracture of the adjacent cribriform plate. Possible cerebrospinal fluid rhinorrhea and pneumocephalous require neurosurgical evaluation.

Orbital Roof Fractures

Fractures of the orbital roof are relatively rare and account for about 5% of facial fractures. The superior orbital rim is broad and well supported and is fractured only by severe blunt trauma as from the impact of a dashboard or steering column in an automobile accident. The roof itself, however, is rather thin and susceptible to penetrating injury. Unilateral forehead anesthesia and decreased frontalis muscle function are clinical signs unique to a frontal sinus fracture. Loss of the first or

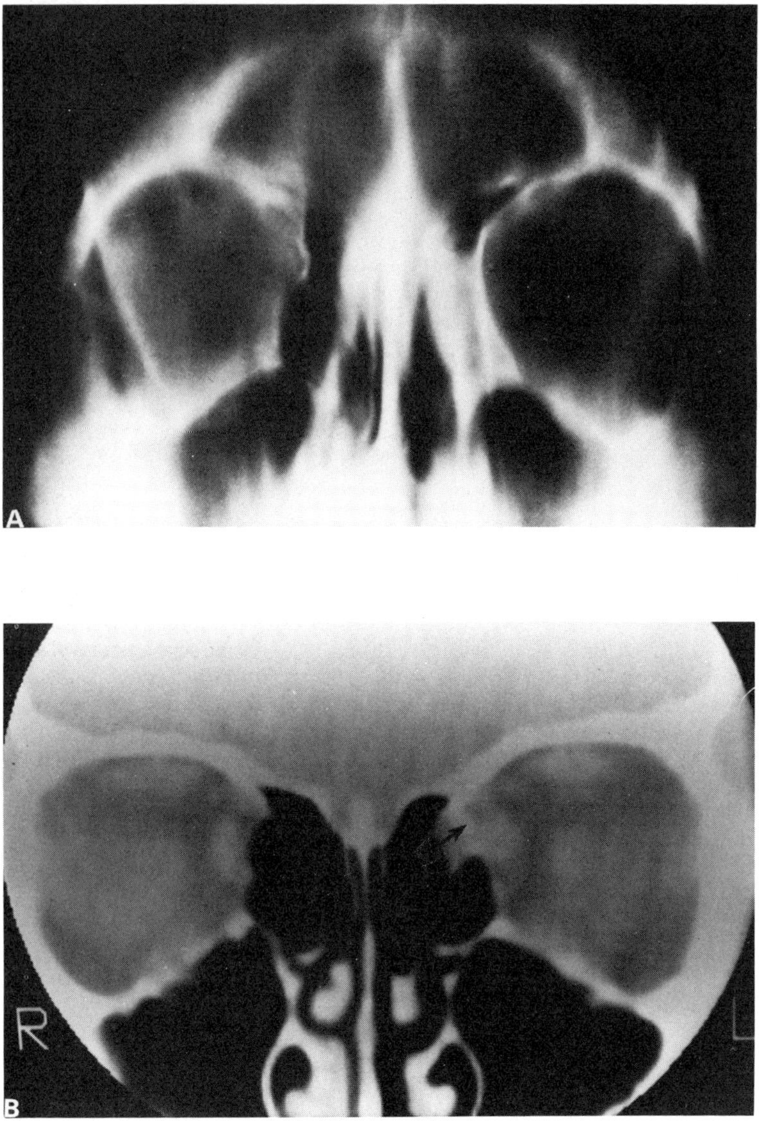

Figs. 8-14A and B. Tomogram (A) shows medial wall fracture. Coronal CT scan (B) shows entrapment of medial rectus muscle (arrow).

second sensory division of the fifth nerve suggests an anterior or middle cranial fossa lesion. Involvement of the petrous portion of the temporal bone may cause facial paralysis or audiovestibular disturbances.

The clinical signs of roof fractures vary somewhat depending on which portion of the roof is fractured. Fractures that occur in the medial aspect of the orbital roof often cause comminuted and depressed fractures of the frontal sinus. Theoretically, fractures in this area may sever the trochlea that support the superior oblique tendon or rupture the medial horn of the levator and cause motility imbalance and ptosis, respectively. Fractures of the supraorbital ridge result in flattening of the brow (Fig. 8-15). Fractures of the lateral roof may disrupt the lateral horn of the levator as it attaches between the palpebral and orbital lobes of the lacrimal gland. Enophthalmos with entrapment of orbital tissues may cause motility disturbances (usually limitation of upgaze). Pseudoptosis may result from depression of the globe. A true ptosis may occur from traumatic neuropathy, or hemorrhage into the levator muscle or its apeneurosis. Entrapment of the levator causing lagophthalmos or lid retraction has not been reported.

Because any orbital roof fracture may be associated with a frontal or ethmoid sinus and cribriform plate fracture, the possibility of a dural tear and pneumocephalous must always be considered. Patients with orbital roof fractures should be evaluated and followed by a neurologist or neurosurgeon. Patients may have meningitis with headache, neck rigidity, changes in the level of consciousness, and ansomnia. Meningitis may lead to frontal lobe abscess formation.

Fractures of the frontal sinus are demonstrated in the P-A and Water's view (Fig. 8-16). The lateral view may be helpful in diagnosing frontal sinus fractures. Posterior wall fractures of the frontal sinus are difficult to demonstrate radiologically, and pneumocephalous may be the only evidence of such a fracture. CT scan is helpful in evaluating orbital roof fractures.

Fractures of the Lateral Wall

The lateral wall or the orbit is unique in that it is the only wall of the orbit that is not at least partially bounded by a sinus. Also unlike the other three walls, entrapment of extraocular muscles has not been reported in association with lateral wall fractures. The bones of the lateral wall are thick and strong.

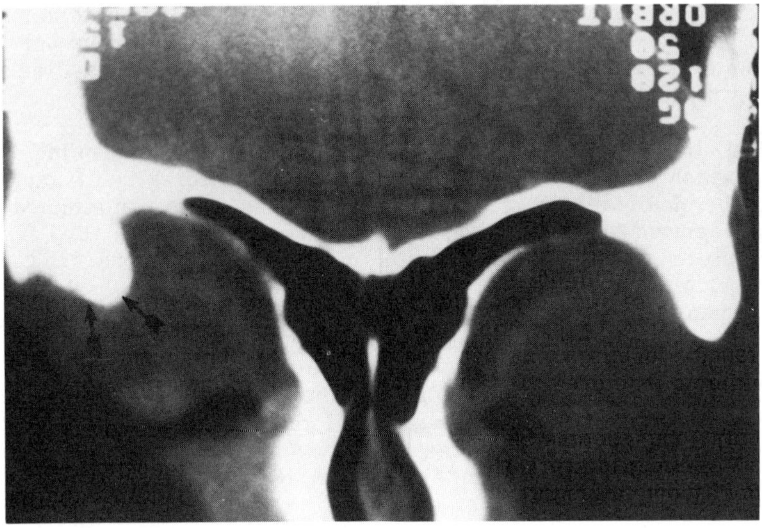

Fig. 8-15. Orbital coronal CT scan shows depressed bony fragments (arrow) of orbital roof. This 28-year-old male was struck with a hammer.

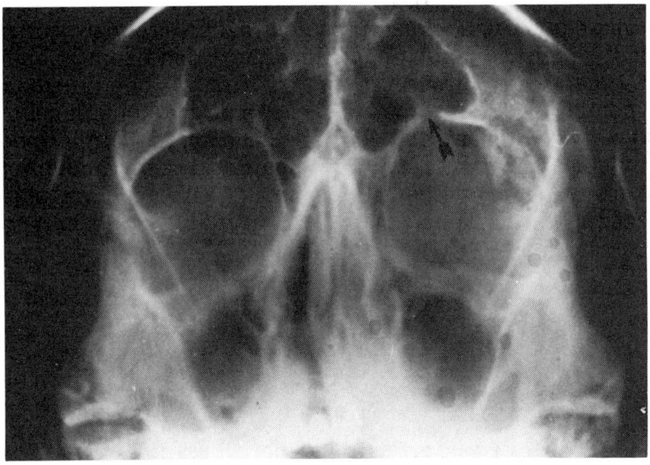

Fig. 8-16. Plain film of orbit (Water's view) shows fracture of orbital roof in area of frontal sinus (arrow).

For this reason, fractures that involve only the lateral orbital rim are rare. It appears that in order to generate a sufficient force to disrupt the lateral wall, an adjacent structure is also injured. The most common combined fractures that involve the lateral orbital wall affect the zygomaticofrontal suture and include tripod fractures and LeFort III fractures.

Combined Fractures

The combination of orbital fractures that can result from trauma is limitless. The types of combined fractures that commonly involve the orbit and/or midfacial structures are considered below as separate entities.

Tripod and Tripartite Fractures

The tripod fracture is caused by direct trauma to the cheek. The three components of the fracture include: (1) separation of the zygomaticofrontal suture, above, (2) the zygomatic arch, laterally, and (3) the zygomatic maxillary suture, medially. The zygoma is usually displaced either backward or downward. The backward displaced zygoma usually results in complete attachment of the zygoma with a step deformity of the inferior orbital rim, a depressed malar eminence, and an elevated zygomatic arch. The fractures that cause downward displacement of the zygoma usually result in incomplete displacement of the zygoma. If the zygoma remains hinged at the zygomaticofrontal suture but detached at the maxillary attachment, the orbital septum will be pulled down and there will be increased scleral show at the lateral aspect of the lower lid. The lateral canthal tendon which inserts at the orbital tubercle 10 mm inferior to the zygomatic frontal suture will remain intact. If the zygoma remains hinged at the zygomatic maxillary suture but detached at the zygomaticofrontal suture, the lateral canthal tendon and the globe will be displaced downward. There will be no increased scleral show.

Most patients with tripod fractures have hypesthesia in the distribution of the second division of the fifth nerve. Malocclusion often develops because of the fracture of the zygomatic arch. Extraocular muscle palsies are rare, probably because the mechanism of the fracture is not that of a blow-out in which orbital tissues are forced through the fracture site.

Radiologically, the basal view is essential in demonstrating discontinuity of the zygomatic bone and arch.

Treatment may be performed by an ophthalmic plastic surgeon, ear, nose, and throat surgeon, or general plastic surgeon. These fractures should be repaired within 2 weeks of the initial injury.

Nasoorbital Fractures

The most frequent cause of nasoorbital fracture is the automobile injury where the patient's face strikes the dashboard or steering column. Because of the anterior to posterior direction of the traumatic force, the nasal bones supported by the nasal spine of the frontal bone and the frontal process of the maxilla push the weaker posterior bones of the medial orbital wall posteriorly. A comminuted fracture of these thinner bones, the lacrimal bone, and the lamina papyracea of the ethmoid results.

The fragments may be displaced along the orbital side of the medial orbital wall, or less commonly, these fragments may penetrate into the ethmoid sinus and produce an out-fracture of the medial wall. In addition, the medial canthal tendon is severed, and the lacrimal sac relationship distorted. Clinically, the patient has a depression over the upper portion of the bridge of the nose, telecanthus, tearing, and epistaxis.

Radiographic views include standard orbital films and tomograms. Dacryocystography may be helpful in demonstrating a lacrimal gland obstruction.

Severe trauma may cause a depressed fracture of the frontal bone, and fracture of the cribriform plate and roof of the ethmoid. As with patients with roof fractures, neurological evaluation for cerebrospinal fluid rhinorrhea and pneumocephalous is indicated.

Nasoorbital fractures are best repaired by an ophthalmologic plastic surgeon and an ear, nose, and throat or general plastic surgeon.

LeFort Fractures

The LeFort fractures (types I, II, and III) all involve the maxilla bilaterally and are predominantly transverse or horizontally oriented fractures. LeFort I (transverse) spares the orbit, while LeFort II (pyramidal) and III (craniofacial dysfunction) involve the orbit. Vertical support to the midfacial bones may explain the horizontal nature of these fractures. As with all orbital fractures, the LeFort fractures represent three of many possible types of combined fractures.

The clinical signs are multiple and include: (1) epistaxis, (2) malocclusion, (3) hypesthesia in the distribution of the infraorbital nerve (LeFort II and III only), (4) ecchymosis, edema, and crepitus, (5) elongation of the midface, and (6) tearing (LeFort II and III only). Of all these possible findings, malocclusion is the most common, and elongation of the midface is probably the most striking. Grasping the upper dental arch allows the motion of the fractured maxilla to be best appreciated.

Radiologically, the Water's projection is optimal for maxillary fractures. P-A and lateral views are sometimes helpful, but often tomography is necessary to demonstrate all the fracture sites. These fractures are described in detail elsewhere.

In summary, the optimal radiologic study is based on the clinical circumstances of the trauma. When multiple facial trauma occurs, tomograms of the orbit and sinuses are the preferred technique of evaluation. When trauma appears limited to the medial and inferior orbital walls, and when there is a possible consequent motility disturbance, the CT scan is best ordered with axial and coronal views to best demonstrate the entrapped extraocular muscle. In cases where the motility is not impaired, tomograms may help to determine the size of the orbital floor fracture better than the CT scan and, therefore, help to predict the likelihood of the patient developing late enophthalmos. In cases where an orbital foreign body is suspected, the CT scan is the most helpful study.

ORBITAL HEMORRHAGE AND ORBITAL CELLULITIS

Blunt trauma may result in extensive hemorrhage with proptosis. X-rays should be obtained to rule out sinus involvement which may lead to secondary orbital infection.

Orbital cellulitis is both a sight- and life-threatening disease. Predisposing causes include trauma, with or without a retained orbital foreign body, sinusitis, and neurosis of an orbital tumor. A history of a dental abscess also may be a predisposing cause. Orbital CT scan is helpful in establishing a cause as well as determining whether an orbital abscess is present or whether there is sinus involvement. Cavernous sinus thrombosis may occur as a sequellae. Intravenous antibiotics should be instituted and the type of antibiotic adjusted based on the results of blood cultures. An intraorbital abscess may need to be surgically drained. Both gram positive and negative organisms are possible. In a child Hemophilus influenzae is also a possibility. In sinus infections and dental abscesses, anaerobes may be considered and appropriate antibiotics started.

PROLAPSED LACRIMAL GLAND

The lacrimal gland has two lobes, a larger superior orbital lobe and a smaller inferior palpebral lobe. Prolapse of either lobe of the lacrimal gland may occur with blunt or penetrating trauma. In the case of a prolapsed orbital lobe, a mass is present in the superior temporal aspect of the upper lid. Repair of the prolapsed orbital lobe is best performed using free needles and a nonabsorbing suture in order to suspend the gland just beneath the superior temporal orbital rim. The surgery is done through a blepharoplasty incision.

ORBITAL FOREIGN BODIES

The history is of great importance in determining the possibility of an intraorbital foreign body. X-rays are indicated in any patient with orbital trauma in whom a foreign body is suspected. Glass may not be demonstrated on routine orbital film unless the glass contains significant quantities of barium or lead (Figs. 8-17A, B, and C). If there is a high clinical suspicion of a glass orbital foreign body, orbital CT scan is extremely helpful. Orbital ultrasound may be of value in localizing small foreign bodies and is helpful where CT is not available.

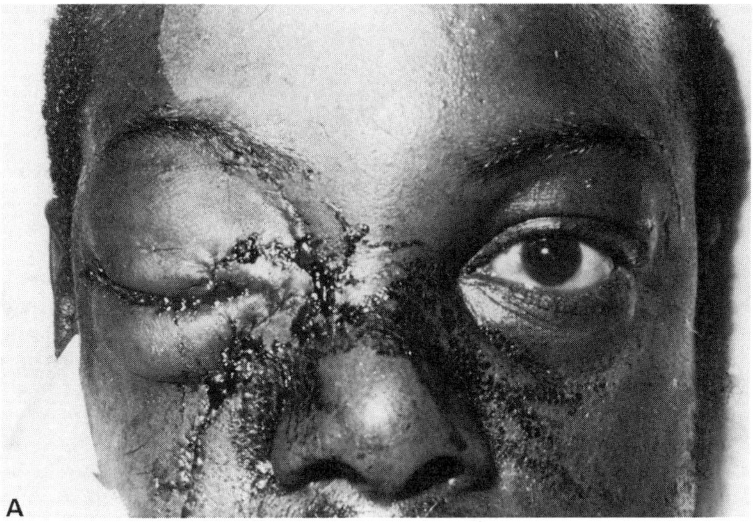

Fig. 8-17A. This 32-year-old male was struck with a beer bottle.

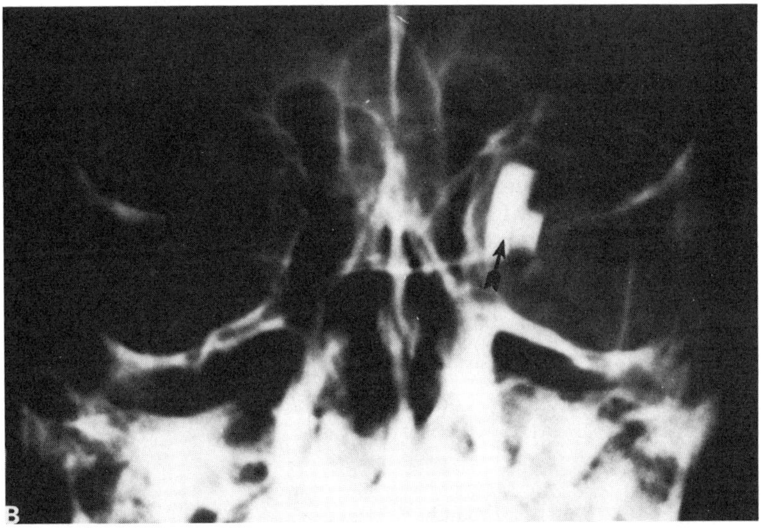

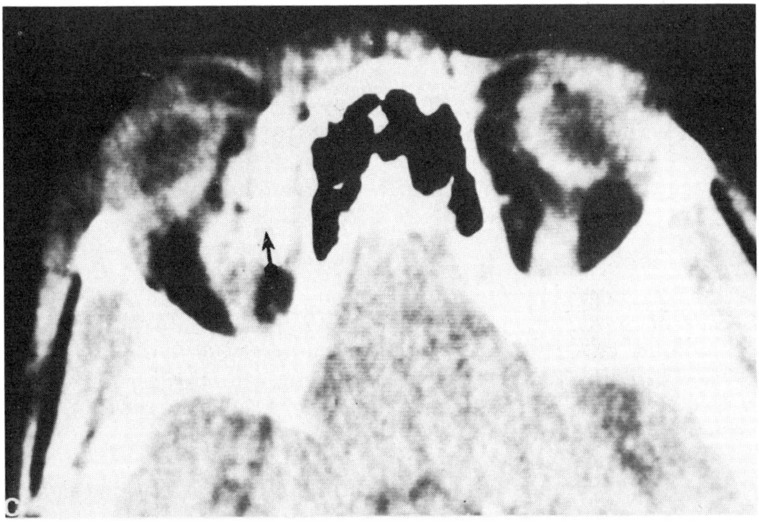

Fig. 8-17B and C. Both plain films (B) and axial orbit CT scan (C) show the presence of a glass foreign body (arrow). Only glass with high lead content, as in this case, will be demonstrated on plain films.

In general, intraorbital foreign bodies are well tolerated and need not be removed. Multiple metallic foreign bodies in the superficial skin are best left. The more superficial ones will gradually surface and the deeper ones need not be removed. Tatooing of the skin occurs at the site of entrance of the foreign body. Dermabrasion may be performed at a later date. Organic orbital foreign bodies should be removed because of the development of a foreign body granuloma and a draining fistula. Plant foreign bodies are often accompanied by infectious processes, including fungi. Metallic, glass, plastic, and lead foreign bodies are probably best left in the orbit unless there is an impairment of visual acuity, ocular motility, or significant secondary inflammatory process (Fig. 8-17A). If a foreign body needs to be removed, the CT scan should be obtained preoperatively and the surgical approach should be through the traumatic site of entry.

BIBLIOGRAPHY

Converse, J. M. and Smith, B.: Symposium: Midfacial fracture, nasoorbital fractures. Trans Am Acad Ophthalmol and Otol 67:622-634, 1963.

Fishbein, F. and Lesko, W. S.: Blowout fracture of the medial orbital wall. Arch Ophthalmol 81:162-163, 1969.

Flanagan, J. C., McLachlan, D. L. and Shannon, G. I.: Orbital roof fractures. Ophthalmology 87:325-329, 1980.

Grove, A., Tadmor, R., Momose, K. and New, P.: Computerized Tomography for Evaluation of Fractures and Foreign Bodies of the Orbit. In Proceedings of the 3rd International Symposium on Orbital Disorders. Amsterdam, September 5-7, 1977. Edited by the Orbital Centre of the Amsterdam University Eye Hospital, Dr. W. Junk Publishers, The Hague, Netherlands, 130-139, 1978.

Jones, I. S.: Symposium: Midfacial fractures x-ray findings. Trans Am Acad Ophthalmol and Otol 67:635-642, 1963.

Schultz, R. C.: In Facial Injuries. Year Book Medical Publishers, Chicago, 126-169, 1970.

Smith, B. and Regan, W.: Blow-out fracture of the orbit. Am J Ophthalmol 44:733-739, 1957.

Zismor, J. and Noyek, A.: Radiographic diagnosis of orbital fractures. In Third International Symposium of Plastic and Reconstructive Surgery of the Eye and Adnexa. S. J. Aston, A. Hornblass, M. A. Meltzer, and T. D. Rees (eds.). Williams and Wilkins, Baltimore, 66-85, 1982.

Chapter 9

STRESS INJURIES

Stress injuries are changes caused by abnormal barometric pressure, sudden variation in barometric pressure, and stress induced by vibration and acceleration.

An increase in atmospheric pressure produces cerebral symptoms because of higher partial pressure of gases in the blood and in the brain tissue and, in that way, causes visual disturbances. The toxic effect starts when the pressure is greater than two atmospheres.

A marked decrease in the barometric pressure results in anoxia. Functional changes in vision are more common than the organic effects. There may be loss in the visual acuity. Dilatation of pupils may be seen. The motor functions of the eyes may be impaired. Disturbances in accommodation and convergence also can be observed. Visual fields can be constricted and the stereoptic vision may be depressed. Vasodilatation of the retinal vessels is among the early signs of anoxia caused by a subnormal barometric pressure. In the hypertensive subject, retinal hemorrhages may appear.

A sudden decrease in atmospheric pressure is the most important factor causing stress injuries. The disease so induced is called Caisson disease. Rapid release of air from the bloodstream forms gas bubbles, causing micro emboli throughout the body. The general symptoms of rapid decompression are varied. Almost every organ can be affected.

Ocular symptoms are not common; however, if they do occur, they are dramatic and serious. Subconjunctival, retinal, or choroidal hemorrhages may occur. Occasionally, the hemorrhage extravasates into the vitreous. Bubbles of gas can be seen in the vessels of the retina. The ophthalmoscopic appearance of central retinal occlusion is present (diffuse edema of the retina and a cherry-red macular spot). Paresis of the extraocular muscles or nystagmus is relatively common. The pupils may become irregular. Functional visual phenomena such as defects in visual fields, flashlights, or complete amaurosis may occur, indicating embolic damage to the intracranial visual pathways and cortex.

Therapy is concentrated on prophylaxis. To prevent serious consequences it is important that the return from abnormal to normal barometric pressure is made gradually. If symptoms persist after return to normal atmospheric pressure, recompression must be undertaken at once and a slower decompression should be achieved.

GRAVITATIONAL AND VIBRATION STRESSES

Modern travel in high-speed airplanes and sudden acceleration or deceleration have introduced stress which may cause visual symptoms. Also, the human body is very sensitive to vibratory and gravitational stress such as is encountered during atmospheric or space flights or when a person is stationed at a piece of machinery for prolonged periods. Rapid vibration, about 40 cycles per second, reduces the visual acuity considerably. Changes in acceleration cause a drop in blood pressure, affecting the blood flow to the head and the eyes. Under these conditions, airplane pilots and astronauts report "greying" of vision. The more severe condition is the "black-out" or sudden and complete loss of vision which may be followed by unconsciousness.

Recovery from a "greying" or "black-out" is rapid. No residual abnormality of the visual system has been observed from repeated "black-outs." Therapy is not indicated in these cases and efforts should be concentrated on prophylaxis.

BIBLIOGRAPHY

Clark, B. and Graybiel, A.: Apparent rotation of a fixed target associated with linear acceleration in flight. Amer J Ophth 32: 549, 1949.

Duke-Elder, S.: System of Ophthalmology, Injuries. Vol. XIV. Henry Kimpton, London, and Mosby, St. Louis, 1972.

Graybiel, A.: Disorientation in pilots. Contact 5:412, 1945.

Symposium of the New Orleans Academy of Ophthalmology. Industrial and Traumatic Ophthalmology. Mosby, St. Louis, 1964.

Vinacke, W. E.: Illusions experienced by aircraft pilots while flying. J Aviation Med 18:308, 1947.

Chapter 10

RADIOLOGY OF OPHTHALMOLOGIC EMERGENCIES

Ancillary tests in ophthalmologic emergencies include: (1) standard radiological views of the orbit, (2) orbital CT scan, and (3) orbital and ocular ultrasonography. Studies such as these are critical in evaluating patients who have a possible intraocular or intraorbital foreign body, fracture of bones, or an inflammatory or neoplastic process involving the orbit or paranasal sinuses. This chapter will help the emergency room physician decide which specific study to order. More detailed information may be obtained by reviewing the orbital section of Chapter 8.

ANATOMY

The orbits are roughly four-sided pyramidal cavities located on both sides of the nasal cavities. The four-sided orbit consists of seven bones. The roof separates the orbital cavity from the anterior fossa of the skull. Anteriorly, the roof is formed by the orbital part of the frontal bone and posteriorly by the lesser wing of the sphenoid bone. The trochlea of the superior oblique muscle is located anteromedially in the frontal bone. The lateral wall of the orbit consists of the greater wing of the sphenoid in its posterior portion. The anterior third of the lateral wall is formed by the zygomatic bone (Fig. 10-1).

The medial wall consists of the following structures, from anterior to posterior: frontal process of the maxillary bone, the lacrimal bone, the lamina papyracea of the ethmoid, and a small part of the body of the sphenoid.

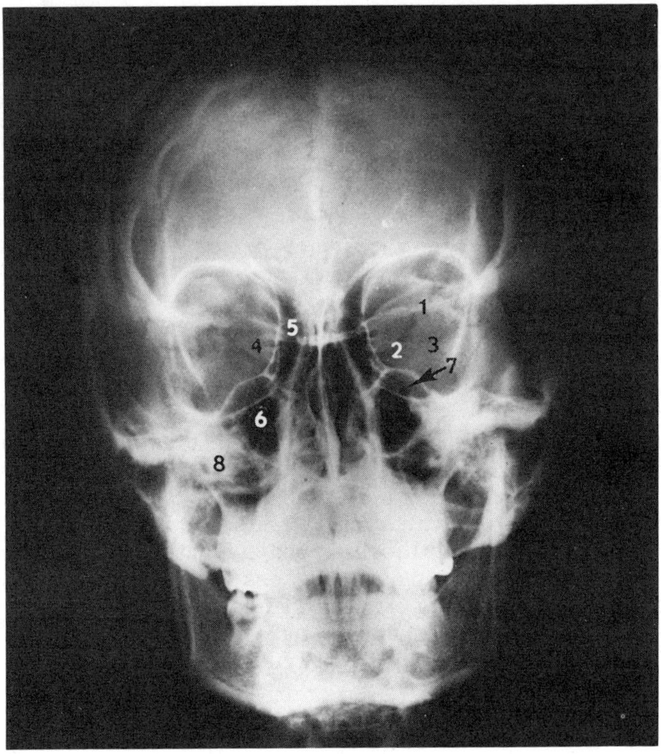

Fig. 10-1. Normal radiographic anatomic appearance of skull. Inside orbital rim, an increased linear density, the sphenoid ridge can be seen (1). Oblique slit is superior orbital fissure (2). Lateral to this radiolucent structure is orbital surface of sphenoidal greater wing forming lateral wall of orbit (3). Superomedial is the lesser wing (4). Medially the dark area is formed by ethmoid cells (5). Below the inferior rim is the maxillary antrum (6). Small hole projected on inferior rim is the infraorbital foramen (7). The petrous bone covers lower third of maxillary antrum (8).

The floor is formed mainly by the orbital plate of the maxilla, the orbital process of the zygomatic bone and posteriorly by the orbital process of the palatine bone. The infraorbital groove is located in the middle of the floor and transmits the infraorbital nerve and its corresponding vessels. The inferior orbital fissure is located between the floor and the lateral wall.

This is known as the sphenomaxillary fissure. The superior orbital fissure is located between the lateral wall and the roof near the apex. Structures which pass through the superior orbital fissure include cranial nerves III, IV, V-1 and VI, sympathetic nerves, arteries, and veins. The optic foramen is located at the apex of the orbit and transmits the optic nerve.

STANDARD RADIOLOGIC VIEWS OF ORBIT

Caldwell View (Fig. 10-2)

This view is a posteroanterior projection of the orbit. This view has the following advantages:

1. The petrous ridges are projected downward and there is a clear visualization of the orbital rim and roof.
2. The greater wing of the sphenoid which forms the majority of the lateral wall is easily detected.
3. The orbital surface of the lesser wing can be seen as projected close to the medial wall.
4. Between these structures—the greater and lesser wings of the sphenoid—the relatively radiolucent slit of the superior orbital fissure is seen.
5. The foramen rotundum is projected under the inferior rim of the orbit.

Water's View (Fig. 10-3)

The main purpose of the Water's view is to obtain a clear view of the maxillary antrum by displacing the image of the petrous bone away from this area. This view is optimal for examination of the orbital roof and most important for evaluation of suspected blow-out fractures in the orbital floor.

Lateral View (Fig. 10-4)

The lateral view is preferable for localization of foreign bodies.

Basal View (Fig. 10-5)

The basal view demonstrates the zygomatic process and is important in patients who have trismus and suspected tripod fractures.

Optic Foramen View (Fig. 10-6)

This view is helpful in evaluating optic nerve tumors and fractures in this area.

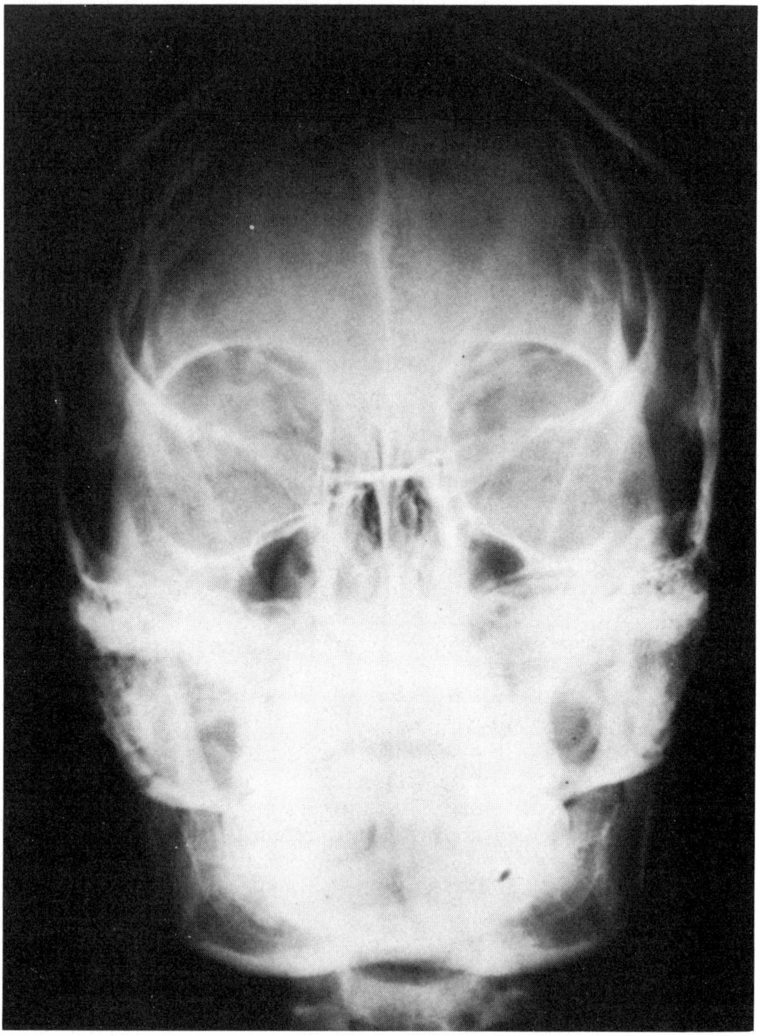

Fig. 10-2. Caldwell view. The orbital rim, orbital roof, the greater and lesser wing of the sphenoid, the superior orbital fissure and infraorbital foramen are visualized in this view.

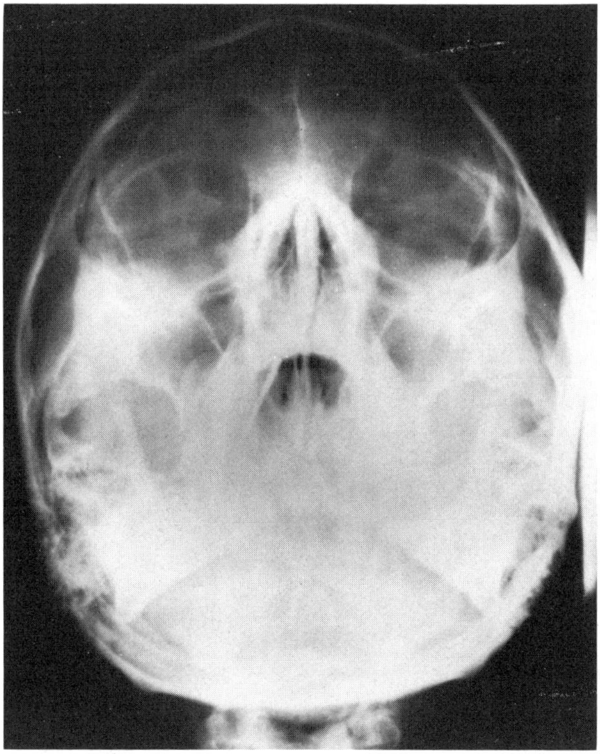

Fig. 10-3. Water's view. The inferior rim, lateral wall of the orbit, superior orbital fissure, zygomatic arch, frontal and ethmoidal sinuses are visualized. The petrous bones are projected downwards and there is a clear visualization of the maxillary antrum.

CHOICE OF STANDARD RADIOLOGICAL VIEWS VERSUS ORBITAL CT SCAN IN EVALUATION OF FRACTURES

In general, plain films of the orbit are adequate for the initial emergency examination in evaluating fractures. The limitation of plain films is that there is generally only one plain of section to demonstrate that a fracture is present. The extent of the fracture is not often well delineated by standard orbital views. In patients with orbital fractures, often a CT scan shows the soft tissue relationship to the fracture and is, therefore, advantageous prior to surgical repair of a fracture. The size of the fracture can be determined only by multiple levels

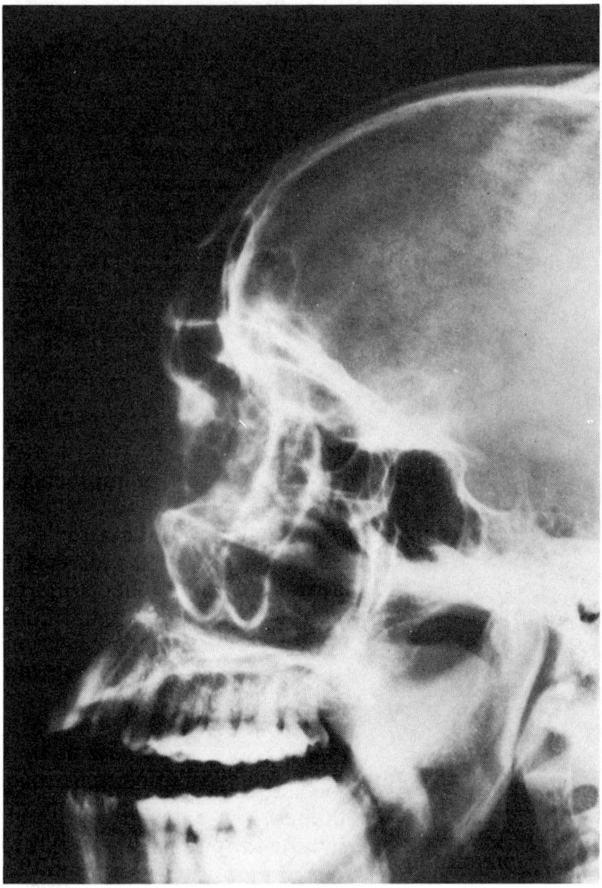

Fig. 10-4. Lateral view of the orbit.

whether by CT scan or orbital tomography. In addition, ethmoidal fractures are very difficult to diagnose on routine films because of the overlapping bones.

In summary, orbital tomography may be substituted for orbital CT scan, but the increased soft tissue detail shown on orbital CT scan makes the latter preferable to orbital tomography.

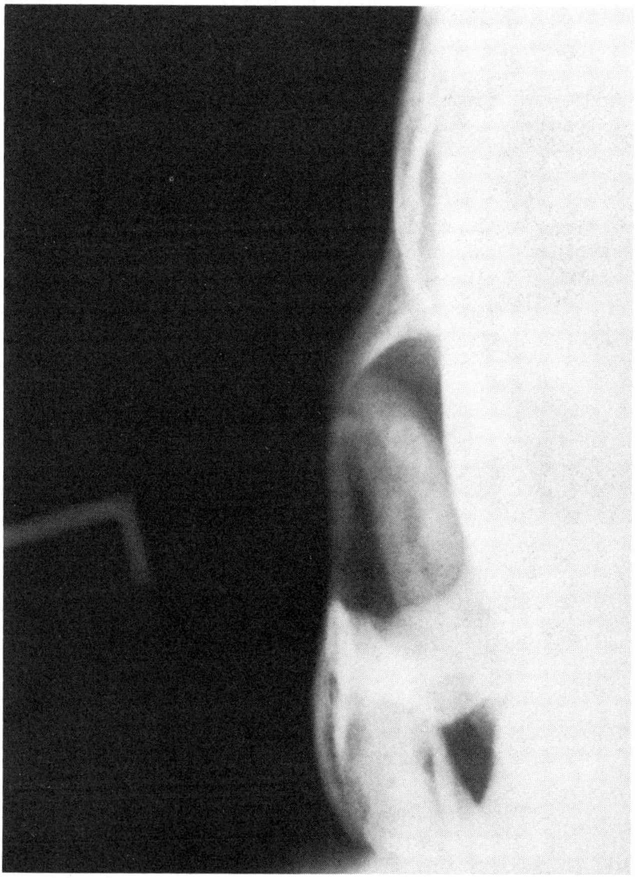

Fig. 10-5. Oblique view, for the external orbital rim and orbital border of the zygomatic bone.

FOREIGN BODIES

Localization of an intraocular foreign body is one of the exact radiological procedures which demands a very accurate study from the radiologist. Unfortunately, it is not possible to differentiate between iron, copper, stone, or lead-containing glass fragments. In general, iron and copper are more radio-opaque than a stone particle, but often the intraocular foreign bodies are so small that their density makes little difference.

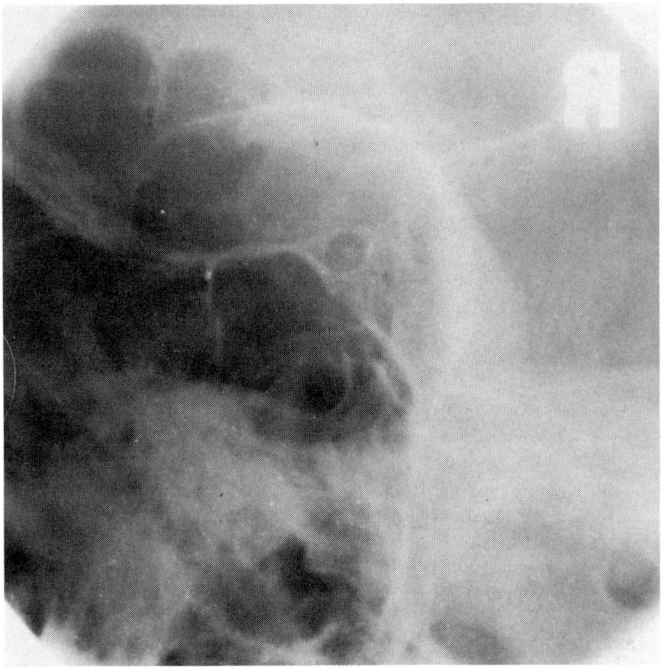

Fig. 10-6. Optic foramen, superior orbital fissure, ethmoid cells, part of the medial wall.

In order to evaluate a possible intraocular foreign body, standard AP and lateral positions are helpful in determining artifact. Calcifications in the area of the lens or a phlebolith, may appear as a possible false positive foreign body.

If it is certain that a foreign body is present in the orbital region, the next step is to determine its accurate location and to find out if the particle is intra- or extraocular. The most common radiologic technique to determine whether an object is intraocular or extraocular is Sweet's method. The equipment consists of a metallic ball and a cone attached to a metallic rod, at a distance of 15 mm. The patient lies on his affected side. The ball is adjusted at a 10 mm-distance from the affected eyeball exactly at the center of the optical axis. Lateral and oblique films are taken and then the localization of the foreign

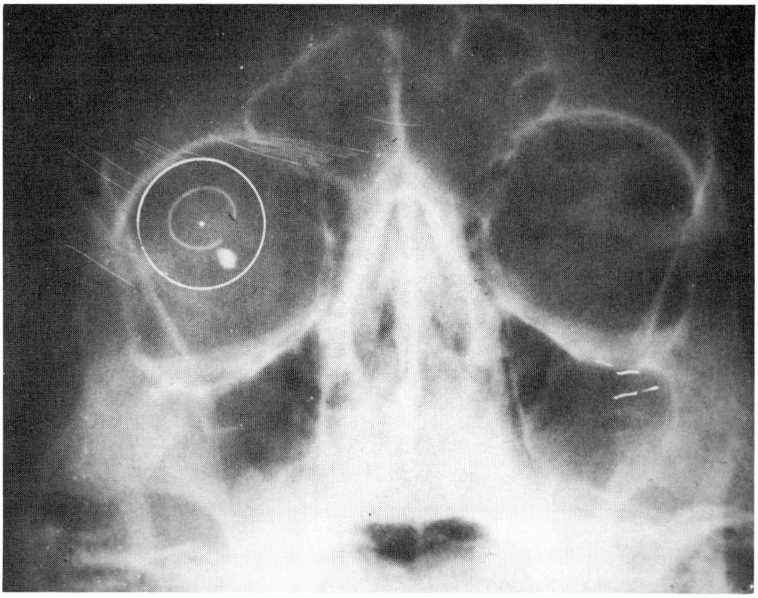

Fig. 10-7. A 25-year-old soldier was wounded by multiple fragments from a hand grenade. His vision deteriorated immediately after injury. Examination of the eyeball revealed suspicious perforation of the sclera and cloudy vitreous. The small circle indicates the metal ring sutured on the corneoscleral border. The outer circle, drawn on the film later, indicates the outline of the eyeball. The increased metallic density between the two circles is the foreign body. The small spot in the center is an artifact.

body is calculated from a specially prepared chart. Another method, the Pfeiffer-Comberg method, uses a contact lens applied on the cornea of the injured eye (Figs. 10-7-10-9). The contact lens contains four built-in opaque dots at 90° intervals indicating the limbus area. PA and lateral exposures will show the location of the foreign body. By drawing in the approximate size of the globe on both films, one can judge whether the foreign body is intraocular or extraocular.

In addition to the radiologic technique discussed above, other methods of identifying foreign bodies, both intraocular and extraocular, include orbital CT scan and ultrasonography. High

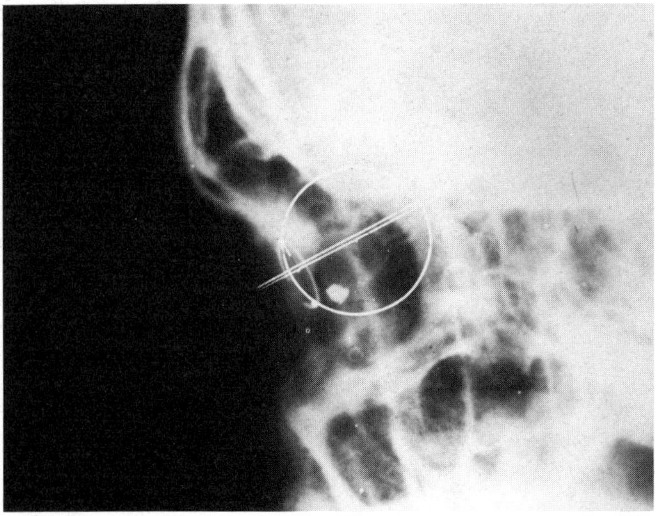

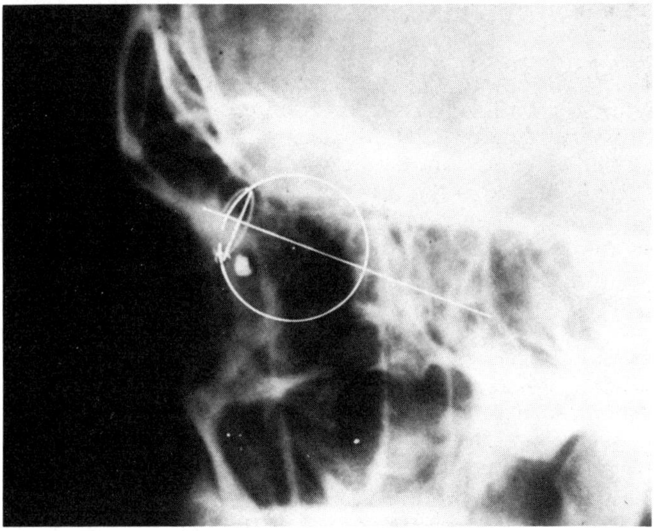

Figs. 10-8 (Top) and 10-9 (Bottom). Lateral view in downward gaze and in upward gaze. The ring sutured on the corneoscleral border indicates the level of the cornea. The drawn circle approximates the outline of the eyeball. The foreign body is intraocular and located anteriorly, since it follows the movements of the eye.

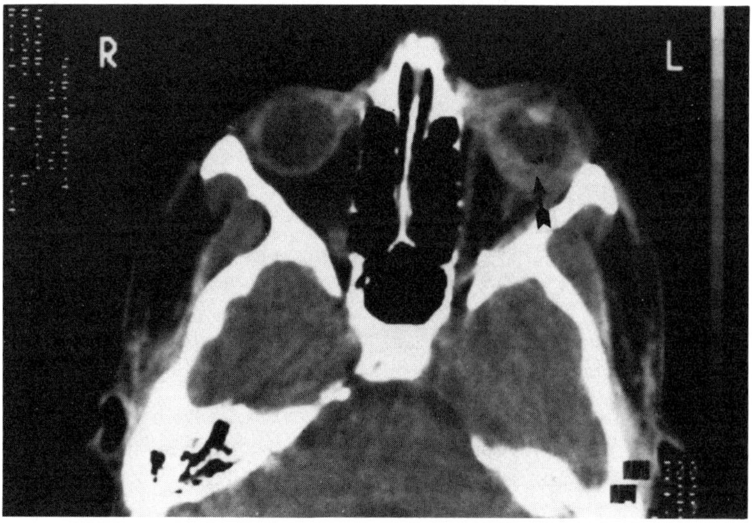

Fig. 10-10. Axial CT scan of the orbit in a patient with a pellet injury to the left eyeball and orbit. Intraocular hemorrhage (arrow) is present.

resolution CT scan may in fact show very minute intraocular foreign bodies and may show detail of evidence of intraocular trauma, including intraocular hemorrhage as well as posterior ruptures of the globe (Fig. 10-10). Orbital ultrasound is a second technique which, in combination with orbital CT scan, may be highly diagnostic and may take the place of other more standard radiologic techniques described above. Either of these techniques will show glass foreign bodies more readily than plain films of the orbit. Only glass with a high lead content can be demonstrated on plain film.

INFLAMMATIONS AND TUMORS

Any inflammation in the orbit or tumor should be evaluated by orbital CT scan. Orbital CT scan will show evidence of bony changes as well as soft tissue changes. Any patient with suspected orbital cellulitis should have a CT scan. Tumors that may masquerade as inflammation may be suspected by orbital CT scan leading to biopsy and definitive diagnosis. In case of a suspected inflammation or tumors, orbital CT should supplant standard plain films of the orbit.

BIBLIOGRAPHY

Bronson, N. R.: Nonmagnetic foreign body localization and extraction. Am J Ophth 58:133, 1969.

Converse, J.M. and Byron, S.: Naso-orbital fractures. Trans Am Acad Ophth & Otolaryng 67:622, 1963.

Dodick, J.M., Berrett, A. and Galin, M.A.: Hypocycloidal tomography and orbital blow-out fracture. Am J Ophth 68:483, 1969.

Merrell, R.A. and Yanagisawa, E.: Radiographic anatomy of the paranasal sinuses. Arch Otolaryng 87:184, 1968.

Pfeiffer, R. L.: Localization of intraocular foreign bodies by means of the contact lens. Arch Ophth 32:261, 1944.

Seymour, E.Q. and Bane, D. B.: A comparison of the accuracy of the Comberg and Sweet techniques of orbital foreign body localization. Radiol 96:75, 1970.

Smith, B. and Regan, W. F.: Blow-out fracture of the orbit. Am J Ophth 44:733, 1957.

Symposium on Radiology of the Orbit. Radiol Clinics of North America 10:No. 1, April, 1972, W.N. Hanafee, ed.

Chapter 11

NEUROOPHTHALMOLOGIC EMERGENCIES

A major portion of the central nervous system is directly concerned with eye function. The afferent system transmits visual information from the retina to the occipital cortex. The efferent system coordinates eye movements and is responsible for pupillary and eyelid control. It is, therefore, common for neurologic disease to present first to an ophthalmologist with primarily ocular symptoms. Neuroophthalmologic evaluation, therefore, requires careful consideration of neurologic as well as ocular disorders.

NEUROOPHTHALMIC EVALUATION

HISTORY

Accurate and thorough history-taking is crucial for proper diagnosis in neuroophthalmology. Visual symptoms must be reviewed in detail. Important features include whether symptoms appeared suddenly or gradually, the character of progression and whether one or both eyes were affected. The duration, frequency, and severity of intermittent symptoms should be reviewed. Associated symptoms (e. g. , pain) must be explored.

A decrease in vision is a major symptom of neuroophthalmologic disease. In monocular visual loss, vision is disturbed in one eye only. A binocular visual disturbance, on the other hand, involves an alteration which affects both eyes. The patient with visual loss should be asked at some point whether he occluded each eye separately to confirm the monocularity or binocularity of visual symptoms. The degree of visual loss may vary from partial to complete. Various patterns of visual field loss may be noted by the patient. "Blurry vision" implies a decrease in central acuity with central scotoma. Patients with homonymous hemianopia may notice that a certain portion of objects appears to be missing. A common observation is that of missing numbers from clock faces. Patients may complain of reading difficulties. Patients with right homonymous hemianopia often have trouble finding the next word on a printed line. The person with a left homonymous hemianopic field cut, on the other hand, can easily locate the next word on a page but has difficulty finding the next line (since this requires seeing on the left side). Patients with bitemporal hemianopia may experience peculiar symptoms such as overlapping of printed words and letters. Words may even appear to slip up and down from one line to the next while reading. A postfixational scotoma may be noted in which there is a zone of absent vision distal to the point of fixation. This occurs in the area where the temporal visual fields overlap when the eyes are to some degree converged.

Another symptom which deserves special discussion is that of diplopia (double vision). Diplopia may be either monocular or binocular. In monocular diplopia, two images of the object of regard are perceived by the involved eye. The second image may be distinct, clear, and separate from the first image. The double image, alternatively, may be less distinct from the primary image and they may largely overlap. This latter form of monocular diplopia is more aptly termed "ghosting." Monocular diplopia results from an optical abnormality in the cornea or lens (e. g. , cataract). Binocular diplopia, on the other hand, results from an abnormality in ocular alignment whereby two different images are perceived simultaneously in the same visual space. Double vision is relieved by occluding either eye. The patient will often spontaneously close one eye or will have already occluded one lens of his glasses. The character of binocular diplopia should be explored, since it may yield clues as to the underlying etiology. First, the patient should be asked whether the two images are displaced horizontally, vertically, or diagonally with respect to each other. Vertical diplopia implies the presence of a deficit in elevation or depression in one eye. Horizontal diplopia, alternatively, may be caused by a relative monocular weakness in abduction or adduction. Diagonal displacement may be caused by some combination of horizontal and vertical imbalance. An inquiry should be made into whether the diplopia is exacerbated by attempted gaze into one particular direction. Image displacement will be maximal when the patient attempts to look into the field of action of the weakened extraocular muscle. For example, a patient with a right lateral rectus weakness will note that the images are wider apart when he attempts to look to the right. The patient should be asked whether the diplopia is greater when he fixates at near or at a distance. Greater difficulty at near (e. g. , while reading) implies an adduction weakness, while worse diplopia with distance fixation (e. g. , while driving) signifies an abduction weakness.

Since many neuroophthalmic problems are related to systemic disease, a thorough past medical history must be obtained. This includes a review of past illnesses, current medications, habits, and a family history.

EXAMINATION

Neuroophthalmic examination begins with determination of a best-corrected visual acuity, either by refraction or pinhole. Color vision is checked with standardized color plates. Visual fields are tested by confrontation (to finger-counting) in all four quadrants of each eye separately. Pupils are examined for their size in light and dark, reactivity to light and near stimuli, and for the presence of a relative afferent pupillary defect (Marcus-Gunn pupil). Ocular alignment, ductions, and versions are observed and the presence of nystagmus is noted. Biomicroscopy of the anterior segment and vitreous is performed and the intraocular pressure measured. Funduscopy is performed with attention to the macula and optic disc. The orbit is examined for the presence of congestion, inflammation, masses, and proptosis.

A brief neurologic examination should be performed. The patient's mental status is checked, noting orientation and alertness. Motor function evaluation should include testing for a pronator drift of the outstretched arms, assessment of extremity strength, and observation of gait. Deep tendon reflexes should be checked and any asymmetry noted. Cranial nerve testing, already largely performed in the ophthalmologic examination, is completed. Evaluation of cerebellar function includes finger-to-nose, rapid repetitive and rapid alternating movements.

AFFERENT SYSTEM

OPTIC NERVE

Optic nerve disease accounts for a major proportion of neuro-ophthalmic emergencies. The hallmarks of optic nerve disease are decreased color vision (dyschromatopsia) relative afferent pupillary defect. Visual acuity is usually diminished. Typical visual field defects include central, paracentral, and arcuate scotomata. The optic disc may appear swollen, pale, or even normal.

<u>Disc Swelling Without Visual Loss</u> (See Appendices III, IV, and V)

Papilledema

Papilledema refers to bilateral swelling of the optic nerve heads caused by an elevation of intracranial pressure. Swelling of the nerve heads secondary to other causes is more aptly described by the general term, "disc swelling." The new diagnosis of papilledema constitutes a neuroophthalmic emergency which requires immediate evaluation.

The patient with papilledema may have a variety of complaints or may even be asymptomatic (see Appendix V). Patients with papilledema may complain of transient visual obscurations. These "blur-outs" are monocular or binocular, last only a few seconds, and tend to be elicited by assuming an upright posture. Symptoms of increased intracranial pressure include headache, nausea, vomiting, and diplopia (due to an associated abducens nerve palsy).

Papilledema progresses through a predictable series of funduscopic changes. Early findings include loss of spontaneous venous pulsations and blurring of the disc margin. Congestion of retinal veins, disc hyperemia, and nerve fiber layer hemorrhages may follow. As the papilledema becomes florid, the disc becomes more elevated (Fig. 11-1), the central cup is lost and nerve fiber layer infarcts (cotton wool spots) are often noted. The nerve fiber layer becomes edematous, obscuring the peripapillary retinal vessels and creating concentric folds of swollen retinal tissue adjacent to the disc (Paton's lines). Although central acuity usually remains normal, perimetry often reveals enlargement of the blind spot and peripheral visual field constriction. In the late stage of chronic papilledema (Fig. 11-2), the disc becomes pale and optic nerve function may decline. An associated ophthalmic finding is sometimes

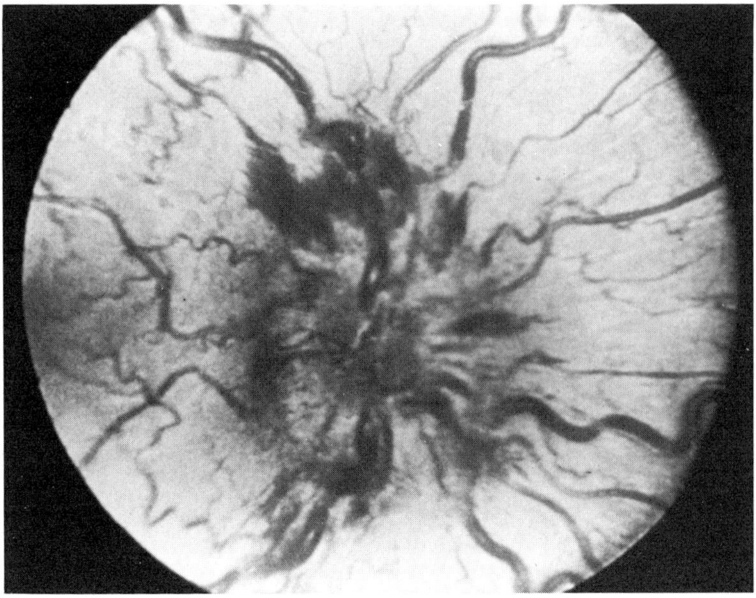

Fig. 11-1. Acute papilledema. (Courtesy, Wills Resident Collection).

that of an abduction deficit; this is due to an abducens nerve palsy which is also caused by an elevated intracranial pressure.

Once the diagnosis of papilledema has been made, an emergency computerized tomographic (CT) head scan is needed to exclude the presence of an intracranial mass. An untreated supratentorial mass may lead to transtentorial herniation with rapidly fatal brainstem compression. Once the possibility of an intracranial mass has been eliminated, then other causes of papilledema should be considered. Appropriate studies include a lumbar puncture with opening pressure measurement to exclude pseudotumor cerebri and meningitis.

Pseudopapilledema

In pseudopapilledema, anomalous fundus changes resemble and may be confused with true papilledema (see Appendix VI). It is important to distinguish this condition from papilledema since it is benign and requires no further diagnostic or therapeutic intervention.

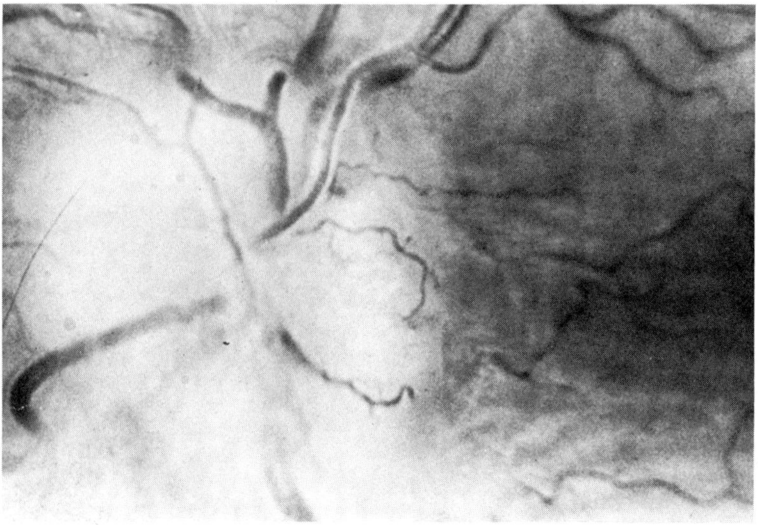

Fig. 11-2. Chronic papilledema. (Courtesy, Wills Resident Collection).

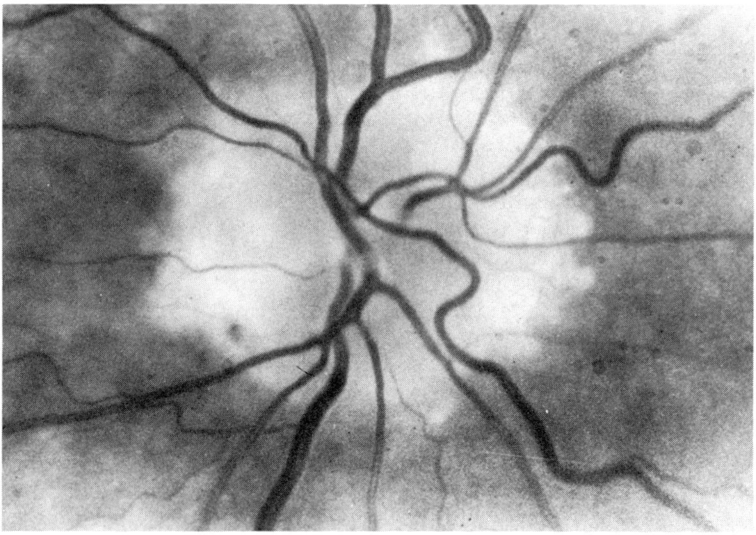

Fig. 11-3. Optic disc drusen. (Courtesy, Wills Resident Collection).

The disc in pseudopapilledema may be elevated secondary to drusen of the optic nerve head (Fig. 11-3). The hyaline bodies may be "buried" or may be ophthalmoscopically visible. As patients become older, buried drusen sometimes enlarge and become apparent on the disc surface. Disc drusen tend to occur in an autosomal dominant pattern; therefore, examination of siblings or parents is helpful. Hemorrhages may occasionally occur on or adjacent to the disc, further complicating the differentiation from true papilledema.

Pseudopapilledema may be distinguished from acute papilledema by a number of features. Spontaneous venous pulsations are usually present. Retinal veins are neither distended nor obscured at the disc margin; the disc is not hyperemic. Disc drusen tend to cause maximal elevation centrally where retinal vessels emerge; thus, the central cup is usually absent. Drusen often cause the disc margin to have an irregular, lumpy appearance. Retinal vessels may appear abnormal with atypical branching patterns and trifurcations. Peripapillary retinal pigment epithelial abnormalities may also be noted.

Disc Swelling With Visual Loss

Anterior Ischemic Optic Neuropathy

Acute anterior ischemic optic neuropathy (ION) occurs in two forms: nonarteritic and arteritic. These are considered separately due to differences in cause, prognosis, and treatment.

Nonarteritic (Idiopathic). In acute nonarteritic ION, the anterior portion of the optic nerve becomes infarcted due to arteriosclerotic, microvascular disease. This optic neuropathy occurs most commonly in the 50 to 65 year-old age group. There may be a history of hypertension or diabetes mellitus. The patient will note the acute onset of painless monocular visual loss, with the appearance of a "smudge" or "haze" over one eye. The visual deficit may worsen over 1 to 2 days but remains fixed thereafter.

Examination will often reveal near-normal visual acuity, although central vision may sometimes drop to 20/400 or to counting fingers. A relative afferent pupillary defect and subnormal color vision are typical features. Pale swelling of the optic disc (Fig. 11-4) is always seen acutely and may occur in a sector fashion. Flame-shaped hemorrhages are also often seen on and adjacent to the optic nerve head. Arcuate or

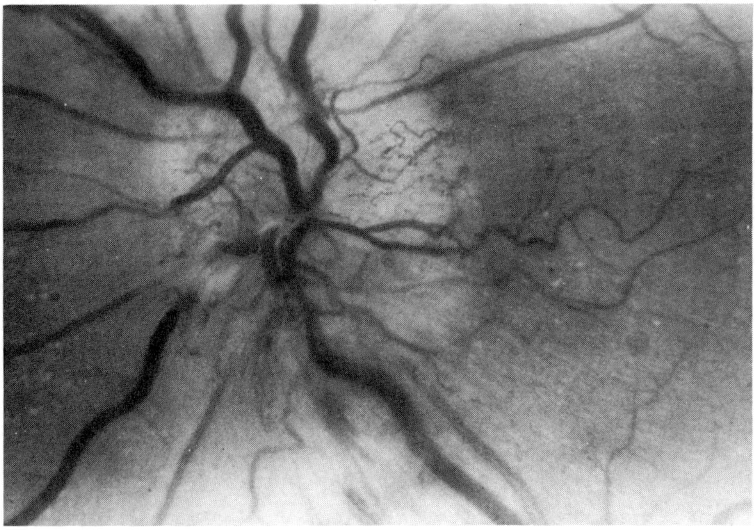

Fig. 11-4. Ischemic optic neuropathy. (Courtesy, Wills Eye Hospital: Neuroophthalmology Unit).

altitudinal visual field defects are typical findings, usually corresponding to the sector of swelling seen on fundus examination. The disc swelling will resolve spontaneously over a period of weeks, leaving some degree of residual optic disc pallor.

Evaluation should include an erythrocyte sedimentation rate to screen for giant cell arteritis. Underlying hypertension and diabetes should be controlled medically. We recommend the use of oral aspirin (1 tablet daily) for its antiplatelet effect. This unproven but safe therapy may be of some benefit in the prevention of a recurrence.

Arteritic (Giant Cell Arteritis, Cranial Arteritis). Giant cell arteritis is a systemic disorder which frequently presents with visual loss secondary to ischemic optic neuropathy. Less commonly, patients with giant cell arteritis may present with acute central retinal artery occlusion. Medium-sized arteries develop inflammation in the vascular wall, causing stenosis of the arterial lumen. Involvement of the ophthalmic blood supply leads to the development of an ION. Occasionally, giant cell arteritis may produce an ischemic third or sixth cranial nerve palsy. Patients with cranial arteritis often complain of headache, scalp tenderness, and jaw claudication. The headache typically has a changing pattern and may be localized over the temporal artery. Patients usually suffer from "polymyalgia rheumatica," a systemic syndrome produced by giant cell arteritis. Symptoms include fever, weight loss, malaise, weakness, and proximal muscle pain.

The arteritic variety of anterior ION is more fulminant than the nonarteritic form and requires immediate evaluation and therapy. Although occasionally seen in patients as young as 55 years, this disorder is primarily a disease of the elderly. The patient will complain of acute progressive monocular visual loss. This may be preceded by several episodes of transient visual loss which simulates amaurosis fugax. It is essential to distinguish this entity from the nonarteritic type, as giant cell arteritis is a progressive systemic disease which is controllable with systemic steroids.

Findings on examination include decreased central acuity on the involved side. Vision tends to be considerably worse than is seen with nonarteritic neuropathy; acuity usually falls in the 20/200 to NLP (no light perception) range. Advanced visual field loss with altitudinal defects is often seen. Fundus examination will reveal typical changes of an ION: pale swelling of the disc, flame hemorrhages and cotton wool spots. Examination of the head may reveal scalp tenderness; swelling and tenderness over the superficial temporal artery may be noted.

Laboratory studies must include an erythrocyte sedimentation rate (ESR) and a complete blood count. The patient with cranial arteritis typically has an elevated ESR, often above 100 mm/hr (Westergen). Since the ESR increases normally with age, 40 mm/hr should be considered the upper limit of normal in the elderly population. Serum protein electrophoresis may reveal elevation of the alpha-1 and alpha-2 globulins. Biopsy of the superficial temporal artery is important to confirm the diagnosis; a negative biopsy, however, does not rule out the diagnosis of giant cell arteritis. Steroid therapy, therefore, should not be withheld in cases where the clinical diagnosis is clear but the biopsy is negative.

Treatment consists of immediate systemic steroid therapy, since 75% of patients with untreated arteritic ION will develop contralateral visual loss. Therapy, therefore, should not be delayed while temporal artery biopsy is being arranged. Patients should be started on 80 mg of oral prednisone daily. Several days of intravenous methylprednisolone (250 mg IV/6 hr) may restore some lost vision if the patient is seen soon after onset of visual loss. Careful inpatient observation is required of patients being treated with intravenous steroids; hyperglycemia and electrolyte disturbances are known potential complications of this therapy. Giant cell arteritis typically remains active for 1-2 years, thus necessitating the use of long-term oral prednisone. Steroids are gradually tapered over 12-18 months; monthly examinations with measurement of the ESR are important to detect exacerbations of arteritis. The complications of long-term systemic steroids are potentially severe and include gastric ulcers, osteoporosis, diabetes, and adrenal suppression. Patients should be followed concurrently by an internist in order to minimize and treat the potential complications of therapy.

Papillitis (Anterior Optic Neuritis)

Papillitis refers to an inflammation of the optic nerve in which the optic disc is involved. The patient will present with a history of progressive visual loss over hours to several days. This may be painless or the patient may experience pain on ductions with ocular tenderness. Examination usually reveals a reduction in visual acuity with a dyschromatopsia and a relative afferent pupillary defect. Biomicroscopy may reveal vitreous cells. Fundus examination will reveal a swollen, hyperemic disc (Fig. 11-5) with fluid in the nerve fiber layer and obscured peripapillary vessels. There may be retinal exudates or a macular star. Hemorrhages may be noted on or adjacent to the disc. Visual field examination will usually show a central scotoma of varying density.

Papillitis usually results from idiopathic inflammation or demyelinating disease (multiple sclerosis). Papillitis may actually herald the onset of multiple sclerosis. A postviral papillitis may follow an upper respiratory infection, probably occurring on an autoimmune basis. Papillitis is occasionally seen as a manifestation of a systemic vasculitis, (e. g. , polyarteritis nodosa) or contiguous paranasal sinusitis. In patients with an atypical presentation or course an ESR, antinuclear antibody titer, and CT scan of the paranasal sinuses should be obtained.

The long-term prognosis for visual recovery with papillitis is

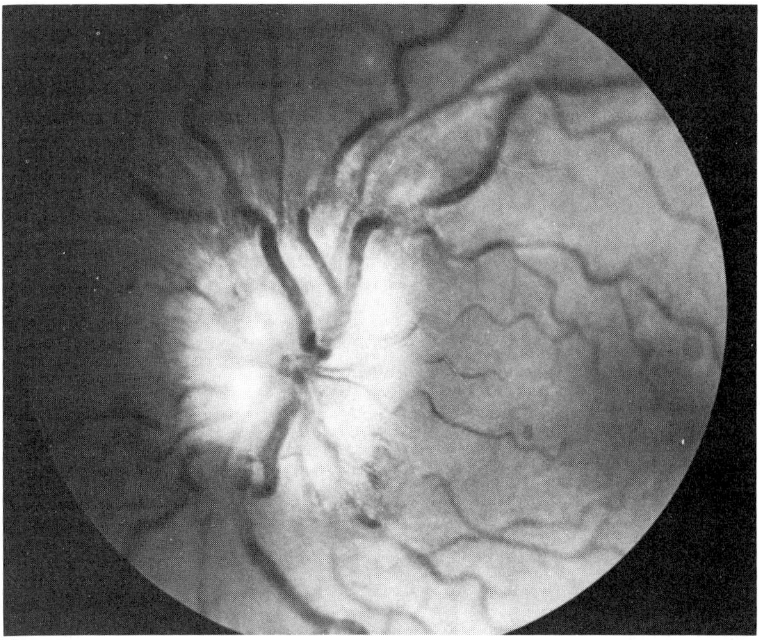

Fig. 11-5. Papillitis. (Courtesy, Wills Eye Hospital: Neuro-ophthalmology Unit).

good. Patients usually experience a gradual return of vision to near-normal over 6 weeks but may continue to improve over 6-12 months. Some degree of disc pallor and a mild dyschromatopsia are typical residual findings. Systemic or orbital steroids appear to reduce the duration of visual loss; it is unclear whether the ultimate visual outcome following papillitis is affected. Monocular patients and the patient with bilateral papillitis may particularly benefit from steroids, as the interval for visual rehabilitation may be considerably reduced.

Other Causes

There are multiple other less common causes for swelling of the optic disc which is associated with visual loss. These include thyroid ophthalmopathy, collagen vascular disease, sarcoid, and meningeal infiltration. When the etiology of a swollen disc with visual loss is unclear, appropriate laboratory tests should be performed to diagnose these other possibilities. Studies may include an ESR, antinuclear antibody titer, CT scan of the orbits and paranasal sinuses, chest x-ray, and lumbar puncture.

Normal Disc With Visual Loss – Retrobulbar Optic Neuropathy

Retrobulbar Optic Neuritis

Retrobulbar optic neuritis is an inflammation of the optic nerve which occurs posterior to the lamina cribrosa. The presentation is similar to that seen with papillitis except that the fundus examination is normal. The patient will describe an acute visual disturbance which progresses over several days and is often associated with pain on ocular movement. Findings include decreased visual acuity, dyschromatopsia, and a central scotoma. One significant difference from papillitis is epidemiologic; retrobulbar neuritis is more commonly seen in adults while papillitis is largely a disease of childhood.

The most common causes of optic neuritis are idiopathic inflammation and demyelinating disease (multiple sclerosis). An acute retrobulbar neuritis may also occur as a manifestation of collagen vascular disease or may occur as an autoimmune phenomenon following viral infection or vaccination. Again, patients with an atypical course should have appropriate laboratory studies to screen for a systemic vasculitis (including ESR and antinuclear antibody titer). Contiguous paranasal sinus infection may also produce the picture of retrobulbar neuritis. The patient may have a history of sinus pain with other evidence suggestive of sinusitis. An evaluation of such patients must include a CT scan of the orbits and paranasal sinuses. Therapy consists of systemic antibiotics with surgical drainage in some cases.

Like papillitis, retrobulbar optic neuritis typically recovers spontaneously over a 4-6 week interval. Visual recovery may be delayed for 6-12 months in some patients. A variable degree of optic disc pallor develops. Frequently, there is mild residual dyschromatopsia even in patients with full recovery of central acuity. Again, visual improvement is probably accelerated by the use of systemic or retrobulbar steroids; the effect of steroids on the ultimate visual outcome is not known.

Compressive Optic Neuropathy

Compressive optic neuropathy occurs as a result of direct external pressure on the optic nerve by an encroaching mass lesion. The patient develops slowly progressive unilateral visual loss which often goes unnoticed for a variable period. The patient then may inadvertently discover monocular visual loss when he occludes the uninvolved eye. Thus, the sudden realization of vision loss must be distinguished from the sudden onset of visual loss. This can often be sorted out when reviewing the history with the patient.

Examination will usually reveal a decreased visual acuity on the involved side. A dyschromatopsia and relative afferent pupillary defect will be seen as well. Fundus examination will reveal some degree of disc pallor. Shunt vessels on the surface of the disc, produced as blood is diverted from retinal veins to the ciliary circulation, are evidence for sphenoorbital meningioma. Visual field changes may include central and arcuate field defects. Contralateral superior temporal hemianopic field loss is very important to detect since it localizes the lesion to the junction with the optic chiasm.

Lesions producing compressive optic neuropathy may affect the nerve in its orbital, canalicular, or intracranial aspects. Underlying causes include meningioma, optic nerve glioma, pituitary tumor, metastatic tumor, and ophthalmic artery aneurysm. Evaluation must include a CT scan with attention to the optic nerves and chiasm to rule out a compressive lesion. Depending upon the individual case, other studies which may be needed include angiography and lumbar puncture. Therapy, of course, will need to be individually planned with surgical decompression being performed when feasible.

Optic Chiasm

The hallmark of chiasmal disease is bitemporal hemianopia which is often associated with unilateral or bilateral decreased visual acuity. Lesions producing a chiasmal syndrome are usually compressive and cause a gradually progressive loss of visual function. The patient will often inadvertently discover a preexisting visual deficit, occluding one eye and then noticing a field defect in the uncovered eye. The patient may then present as an emergency, with sudden realization of visual loss.

Examination will reveal a variable degree of decreased acuity and dyschromatopsia. A relative afferent pupillary defect will be seen if optic nerve involvement is asymmetric. Optic disc pallor is characteristic. Visual fields by confrontation to finger-counting may reveal a temporal field defect; relative desaturation of the color red in the temporal hemianopic field is a more consistent finding. Formal perimetry will reveal some degree of a unilateral or bilateral temporal hemianopic field cut along with unilateral or bilateral changes of optic neuropathy. Evaluation must include a CT scan of the sella and suprasellar space.

Lesions producing chiasmal dysfunction include pituitary adenoma, craniopharyngioma, glioma, meningioma, and aneurysms of the internal carotid artery. Pituitary adenoma (Fig. 11-6) is the most common compressive lesion of the chiasm, with prolactinoma being the most frequent type. Symptoms of pituitary tumor among women include amenorrhea and galactorrhea. Treatment modalities include systemic Bromocryptine, surgical decompression, and radiation therapy. Before undergoing general anesthesia, the patient should have a thorough preoperative endocrinologic evaluation for possible panhypopituitarism. Thyroid studies and a cortisol level should be obtained.

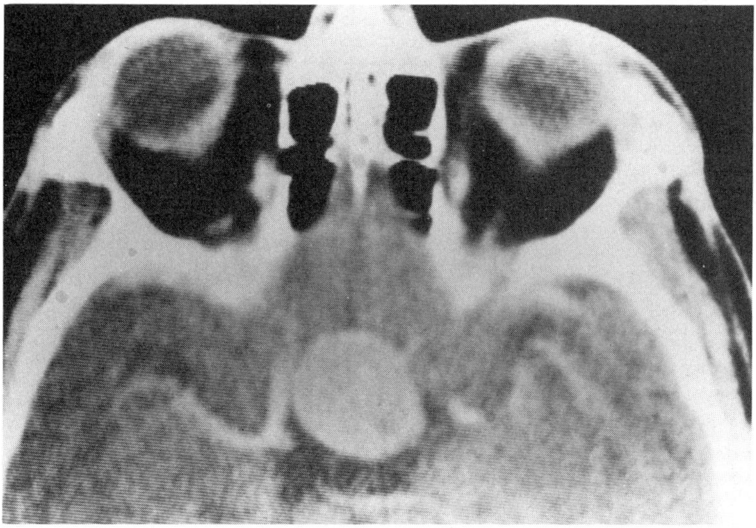

Fig. 11-6. Computerized tomography showing a pituitary adenoma.

Pituitary apoplexy may present with a syndrome of acute, severe visual loss. Apoplexy occurs as a result of necrosis and bleeding into a preexisting pituitary tumor. The patient may have acute or subacute visual loss, diplopia, and headache. Findings on examination will reveal a variable degree of unilateral or bilateral visual deficits. Asymmetric optic nerve involvement may produce a relative afferent pupillary defect. Visual field changes include that of a unilateral or bilateral optic neuropathy with a variable, superimposed bitemporal hemianopic field defect. Evaluation of patients with suspected pituitary apoplexy requires emergency CT scanning of the head with attention to the sella and parasellar areas. Patients with progressive visual loss may require an emergency craniotomy with decompression of the chiasm and optic nerve. It must be remembered that these patients often have secondary adrenal insufficiency and may require systemic corticosteroids, especially if general anesthesia is being contemplated.

OPTIC TRACT

Disease of the retrochiasmal visual system produces homonymous hemianopia. The pattern of field loss is variable and depends upon the area affected. Lesions of the optic tract will very rarely present as an emergency with acute visual loss. Optic tract dysfunction is usually produced by compressive mass lesions, such as craniopharyngeoma or carotid aneurysm. Findings will typically include decreased visual acuity, decreased color vision, and an incongruous homonymous hemianopia. A contralateral relative afferent pupillary defect may be noted because more than half of the pupillomotor fibers decussate in the optic chiasm. Evaluation of these patients must include computerized tomography.

OPTIC RADIATIONS

Lesions of the optic radiations also result in homonymous hemianopia. This type of visual field deficit is most frequently caused by cerebrovascular disease, although mass lesions are not uncommon. Transient visual changes with associated neurologic symptoms which spontaneously resolve are characteristic of transient ischemic attack. A persistent cerebral deficit, on the other hand, suggests infarction.

Parietal lobe lesions tend to produce a homonymous hemianopia which is denser inferiorly and may appear as an inferior homonymous quadrantanopsia. Concomitant neurologic findings often include hemiparesis, aphasia, apraxia, agnosias, right-left confusion, and sensory loss. Temporal lobe disease, on the other hand, tends to produce a homonymous hemianopia which is denser superiorly (the "pie in the sky" defect).

Patients with transient ischemic attacks producing visual changes and other neurologic symptoms require immediate referral to a neurologist for evaluation. The presence of a persistent deficit indicates probable cerebral infarction. Evaluation must include an emergency CT scan; hospital admission is usually indicated for observation and treatment. A progressive, nonhemorrhagic infarction may respond favorably to systemic anticoagulation. Patients with cerebral infarction should be evaluated for the presence of an embolic source.

OCCIPITAL CORTEX

Lesions of the occipital cortex usually produce a highly congruous homonymous hemianopia. Unlike lesions affecting the optic radiations, disease of the occipital lobe may produce a homonymous hemianopia without any evidence of other neurologic signs or symptoms. The principal causes of occipital dysfunction are cerebrovascular disease and, less commonly, mass lesions. Symptoms which resolve spontaneously over minutes to hours indicate probable transient ischemic attack; persistent visual deficits suggest occipital lobe infarction. Examination will usually reveal a normal visual acuity. Formal perimetry will show a highly congruous homonymous hemianopia with "macular sparing." Involvement of the occipital tip may result in homonymous hemianopic paracentral scotomas. These patients should be referred immediately to a neurologist for evaluation. Diagnostic studies must include a CT scan of the head. Again, an embolic source should be considered in cases of cerebral infarction.

EFFERENT SYSTEM

SUPRANUCLEAR PATHWAYS

A detailed discussion of the supranuclear control of eye movements is beyond the scope of this chapter. Several syndromes are discussed which may include an acute motility disturbance secondary to supranuclear pathway involvement.

Gaze Palsy

Frontal Lobe

Fibers which control voluntary horizontal eye movement originate in the premotor cortex of the frontal lobe and descend through the internal capsule to the contralateral pons. Control is exerted over contralateral horizontal eye movement. The right frontal lobe, therefore, controls eye movement to the left; the left frontal lobe, movement to the right. Cerebrovascular disease involving the frontal lobe may produce a neurologic syndrome which includes the finding of a horizontal gaze palsy. The patient with frontal lobe infarction will typically develop a weakness in horizontal versions away from the side of the lesion. Thus, a contralateral gaze palsy results. Other findings typically include a hemiparesis on the same side as the gaze palsy (contralateral to the lesion). These patients, of course, need neurologic evaluation and appropriate rehabilitative care. Gaze palsy following frontal lobe infarction typically clears several days after the cerebrovascular event even though other neurologic deficits may persist.

Pons

Pontine lesions may also result in a disturbance of horizontal gaze. The parapontine reticular formation (PPRF) controls ipsilateral horizontal gaze through connections with the ipsilateral lateral rectus (directly to the sixth nerve) and the contralateral medial rectus (indirectly through the medial longitudinal fasciculus to the oculomotor nerve).

Pontine infarction produces an ipsilateral defect in horizontal gaze (toward the side of the lesion). Other findings typically include an ipsilateral facial nerve palsy and a contralateral hemiparesis. This is to be contrasted with hemispheric disease in which the gaze palsy is on the same side as the hemiparesis. Patients with signs of acute pontine stroke need an emergency neurologic evaluation, which includes a CT scan and hospital admission for observation.

Internuclear Ophthalmoplegia

Internuclear ophthalmoplegia (INO) results from disease of the medial longitudinal fasciculus (MLF) in the brainstem. The MLF is a paired paramedian collection of fibers which interconnects the parapontine reticular formation with the contralateral medial rectus subnucleus of the oculomotor nerve. Each side of the paired MLF controls adduction of the ipsilateral eye. A lesion involving the right MLF will produce adduction deficit of the right eye; this is referred to as a right INO. Abducting nystagmus of the contralateral eye is also seen.

An INO may result either from generalized brainstem disease (with other neurologic findings) or may occur as an isolated finding due to a discrete lesion involving the MLF. The patient will typically note the sudden onset of horizontal diplopia which is made worse on gaze away from the side of the lesion. There are two main causes of an acute INO: brainstem infarction and demyelinating disease (multiple sclerosis). In brainstem infarction, the typical finding is that of a unilateral INO (on the side of the lesion). This is due to the fact that small perforating arteries provide a separate blood supply for each side of the paired MLF. Thus, an infarction may occur in the distribution of one small perforator which causes MLF dysfunction on one side while leaving the other side intact. Demyelinating disease, on the other hand, tends to produce a bilateral INO (Fig. 11-7). Demyelinating lesions usually involve both sides of the MLF (which are anatomically juxtaposed in the brainstem). Patients with an INO require a careful neurologic evaluation. Both demyelinative and vascular types of INO tend to spontaneously resolve. Like optic neuritis, an INO may occur in patients with preexisting demyelinating disease or may alternatively herald the onset of multiple sclerosis.

Two other brainstem disorders with INO should be mentioned. Bilateral INO may occur which presents with a large exotropia in primary gaze and has been termed the "WEBINO" (wall-eyed bilateral INO) syndrome. Bilateral abducting nystagmus is also typically noted. The "one and one-half" syndrome is a second brainstem disorder of interest. In this variant, there is a lesion of the parapontine reticular formation with ipsilateral MLF involvement. This causes a gaze palsy with an INO ipsilateral to the side of the lesion. The only horizontal eye movement left intact is abduction of the contralateral eye. This syndrome is typically caused by brainstem infarction; concomitant ipsilateral facial weakness and contralateral hemiplegia are usually seen.

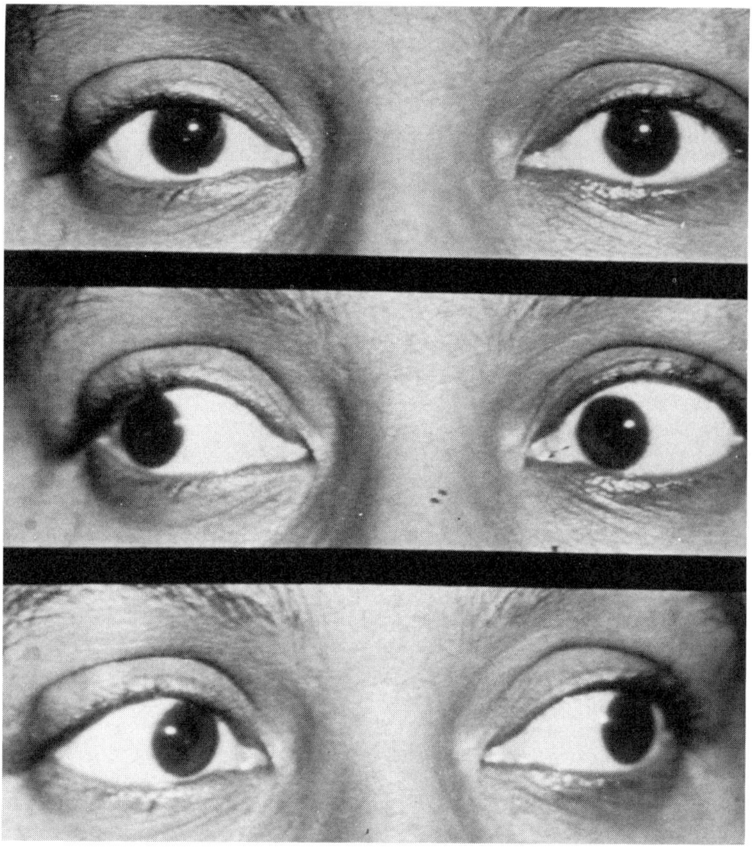

Fig. 11-7. Internuclear ophthalmoplegia. (Courtesy, Wills Eye Hospital: Neuroophthalmology Unit).

CRANIAL NERVE PALSY

Oculomotor Nerve

The oculomotor nerve can be affected by disease involving its nuclear, fascicular, or peripheral segments. The third nerve nuclei are paired midbrain structures which give rise to fibers forming the fascicular portion. The peripheral oculomotor nerve then exits anteriorly into the interpeduncular fossa, coursing forward through the subarachnoid space. The nerve passes through the cavernous sinus and divides into superior and inferior divisions just before entering the orbit through the superior orbital fissure. Structures innervated by the superior division consist of the superior rectus muscle and the levator palpebrae. The inferior division supplies the medial rectus, inferior rectus, inferior oblique, and pupillary sphincter muscles. Oculomotor palsy, therefore, includes the findings (Fig. 11-8) of upper lid ptosis, ophthalmoparesis (deficient elevation, adduction, and depression), and a mydriatic, hyporeactive pupil. Selective lesions involving the superior or inferior division may cause deficits in the distribution of the involved branch.

Brainstem disease can cause oculomotor palsy by involving its nuclear and fascicular portions. Acute brainstem lesions producing third nerve palsy include various infarction syndromes and present with other neurologic findings. In Benedikt's syndrome, structures affected include the oculomotor nucleus, red nucleus, and corticospinal tract. Findings will include oculomotor palsy, contralateral ataxia, and contralateral hemiparesis. Weber's syndrome is caused by an infarction of the ventral midbrain with involvement of the fascicular oculomotor nerve and the cerebral peduncle. The patient will typically present with an ipsilateral third nerve palsy and contralateral hemiparesis.

Acute peripheral oculomotor palsy will present with binocular diplopia and upper lid ptosis. Examination will reveal weakness of those structures supplied by the third cranial nerve. The nerve can be affected at any point in its course; other physical findings will help localize the causative lesion. Acute isolated oculomotor palsy is a fairly common emergency which deserves special discussion. Some motor functions of the oculomotor nerve may be affected more than others; the pattern of oculomotor palsy is extremely important in determining the underlying etiology. The two most important syndromes are microvascular infarction and compression by a posterior communicating artery aneurysm.

Microvascular infarction of the oculomotor nerve occurs most commonly in diabetic patients but also may be seen in hypertensives and those with known vascular disease. The patient with a vasculopathic third nerve palsy presents with the acute onset of upper lid ptosis and binocular diplopia. Ocular and orbital pain will often occur either as a prodrome or concomitant with the onset of third nerve palsy. The degree of ophthalmoparesis varies from mild to complete paralysis of the

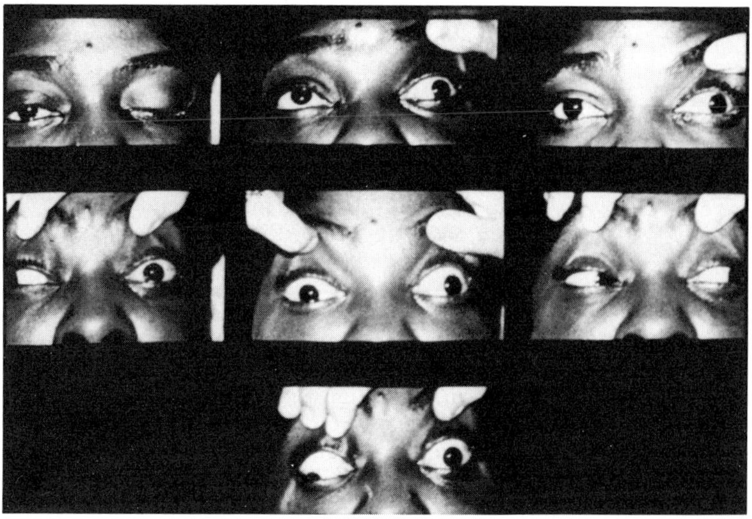

Fig. 11-8. Oculomotor palsy. (Courtesy, Wills Resident Collection).

extraocular muscles supplied by the oculomotor nerve. Upper lid ptosis is also variable but tends to parallel that of motility changes. The pupil typically is "relatively spared." This means that there is only mild anisocoria and pupillary hyporeactivity; the pupil is always affected to a much lesser degree than that of other structures supplied by the oculomotor nerve. If the degree of pupillary involvement parallels that of ophthalmoparesis and ptosis or if the pupil is quite dilated and only barely reactive, then a compressive etiology of the oculomotor palsy must be strongly considered. Microvascular oculomotor palsy may be the presenting sign of previously undiagnosed diabetes mellitus; evaluation of a pupil-sparing neuropathy should include a fasting blood glucose. Blood pressure, of course, should be checked and hypertension treated. Elderly patients can occasionally present with an oculomotor palsy as a manifestation of giant cell arteritis; an erythrocyte sedimentation rate is appropriate in the evaluation of these patients. The prognosis for recovery of oculomotor function is good. Normal third nerve function usually returns over a period of 6-12 weeks.

Aneurysms of the posterior communicating artery are known to produce compressive oculomotor palsy with involvement of the pupil. The patient may present with severe headache and an acute, complete oculomotor palsy. The pupil is typically fixed and dilated. Subarachnoid hemorrhage may cause a decreased level of consciousness or coma. An acute compressive third nerve palsy represents a neurosurgical emergency and requires immediate evaluation. Studies include a CT scan and carotid angiography to rule out a posterior communicating aneurysm. Craniotomy and clipping of the aneurysm are then undertaken to prevent the impending aneurysmal rupture.

Another important cause of peripheral oculomotor palsy is transtentorial herniation. In this syndrome, a space-occupying mass above the tentorium causes a physical shift of the medial temporal lobe (uncal gyrus) through the tentorial opening. The herniating uncus may press the oculomotor nerve against the petroclinoid ligament, causing a compressive palsy. Subsequent brainstem compression produces a loss of consciousness and respiratory arrest. Oculomotor palsy secondary to uncal herniation is said to precede brainstem compression. In a patient with a progressive supratentorial mass (e. g. , subdural hematoma), the onset of an oculomotor palsy may warn of impending brainstem compression. Such patients need immediate medical therapy to reduce intracranial pressure followed by neurosurgical decompression.

There are multiple other causes of acute oculomotor palsy, including head trauma, meningitis, cavernous sinus aneurysm, or tumor, and carotid-cavernous fistula. The acute onset of a third nerve palsy requires immediate evaluation since it may signal a potentially serious underlying neurologic problem. On the other hand, recognition of oculomotor palsy caused by a benign condition (e. g. , vasculopathic) may spare the patient unnecessary and often invasive diagnostic procedures.

Trochlear Nerve

The trochlear nerve arises from paired nuclei in the periaqueductal gray matter caudal to the oculomotor nuclei, courses dorsally to exit the brainstem, and then decussates in the anterior medullary velum. After encircling the brainstem, it penetrates the dura, traverses the cavernous sinus, and enters the orbit through the superior orbital fissure to supply the superior oblique muscle. The trochlear nerve is the longest cranial nerve and is the only one which leaves the brainstem posteriorly.

Patients with acute fourth nerve palsy typically complain of vertical binocular diplopia. Actions of the superior oblique include depression, intorsion, and abduction. Findings on examination will include an ipsilateral hypertropia which increases on contralateral gaze and on tilting the head towards the involved (hypertropic) eye. Patients often tilt their heads spontaneously away from the lesion in an effort to lessen the hypertropia and improve the diplopia. Testing with a double Maddox rod will reveal excyclotorsion of about 5°.

The most common etiology of acute trochlear nerve palsy is head trauma. Head injury with shifting of the cranial contents is thought to damage the fourth nerve where it crosses the tentorial edge. Trochlear nerve function may recover spontaneously; some patients may require eye muscle surgery, however, to correct a persistent hypertropia and excyclotropia.

Simultaneous bilateral trochlear nerve palsy may also occur as a result of head trauma. Damage is thought to occur in the anterior medullary velum (dorsal brainstem) where the trochlear nerves cross in the subarachnoid space. Such patients may be seen to have a left hypertropia on left gaze, V-pattern esotropia, and excyclotorsion of greater than 8°. It is important to recognize bilateral neuropathy in order to plan an appropriate surgical procedure for correction of hypertropia and excyclotropia.

Abducens Nerve

The abducens nerve arises from the brainstem nuclei in the floor of the fourth ventricle and exits the pons anterolaterally at the pontomedullary junction. It then ascends on the pons, penetrates the dura on the clivus, and passes through the cavernous sinus. The sixth nerve then enters the orbit through the superior orbital fissure where it supplies the lateral rectus muscle.

The patient with an abducens nerve palsy will complain of horizontal binocular diplopia which increases on attempted gaze toward the involved eye. Examination will reveal an abduction deficit of the paretic eye; this may be only partial with a decreased saccadic velocity on abduction or may be complete with an inability to abduct beyond the midline. An incomitant esotropia will be noted which is greatest on ipsilateral gaze (Fig. 11-9).

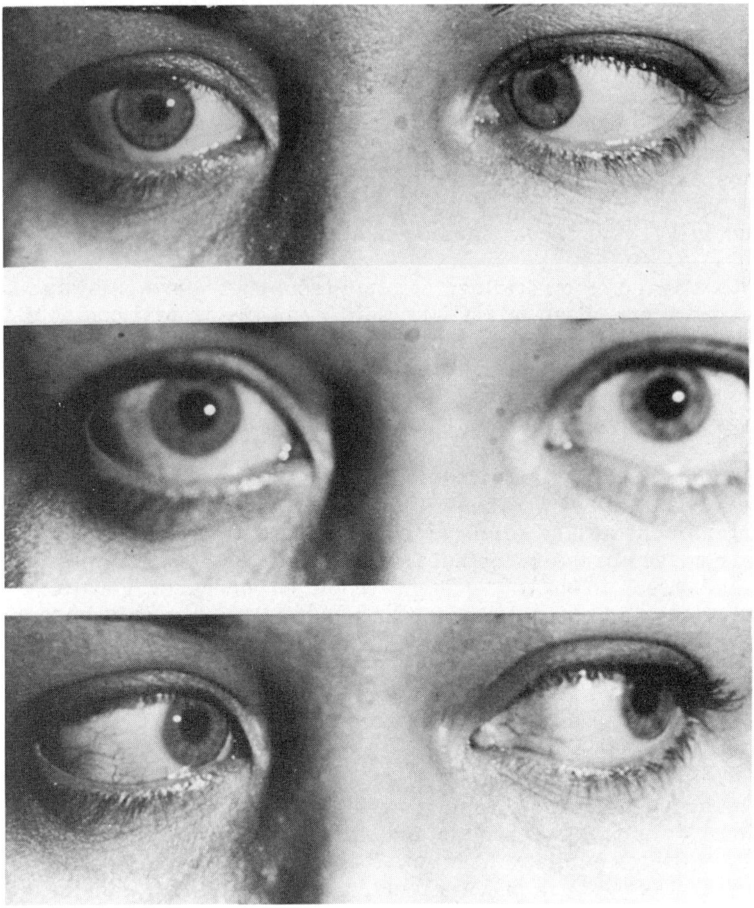

Fig. 11-9. Abducen's palsy. (Courtesy, Wills Resident Collection).

Various brainstem syndromes can involve the abducens nerve in its nuclear and fascicular portions. The two most common etiologies are vascular and demyelinating disease. Adjacent structures which are often involved include the fascicular facial nerve, MLF, PPRF, and corticospinal tract. The finding of multiple neurologic deficits localizes the underlying lesion to the brainstem. The Millard-Gubler syndrome is produced by pontine infarction; findings include ipsilateral abducens and facial palsies with contralateral hemiplegia. Any patient with a suspected brainstem syndrome requires an immediate neurologic consultation for evaluation and treatment. Appropriate studies will include a CT scan to detect brainstem stroke or underlying tumor.

Peripheral abducens palsy may be produced by lesions anywhere between the brainstem and orbit. Microvascular neuropathy is the most common cause of acute isolated peripheral sixth nerve palsy. Patients are usually older than 50 years and often have a history of diabetes mellitus or hypertension. As in third and fourth nerve palsies, a microvascular neuropathy has a good prognosis and usually improves spontaneously within 4-6 weeks.

Increased intracranial pressure may produce a sixth nerve palsy; this is thought to occur as a result of stretching the nerve as the brainstem is shifted caudally. Other symptoms of intracranial hypertension (headache, dizziness, etc.) are often present; fundus examination usually reveals signs of papilledema. Such patients must have an emergency CT head scan to rule out an intracranial mass.

Other causes of abducens palsy are multiple and include paraviral autoimmune neuropathy, basilar meningitis, and multiple sclerosis. Tumors causing sixth nerve palsy can arise in the cerebellopontine angle, clivus, nasopharynx, pituitary, and cavernous sinus.

The evaluation of abducens nerve palsy depends upon the patient's age, previous history, and the presence of other neurologic findings. Patients older than 50 years with an "isolated" nerve palsy (no other neurologic symptoms or deficits, no history of tumor or neurologic disease) should be presumed to have a microvascular neuropathy. Blood pressure should be measured and a fasting blood glucose obtained. An erythrocyte sedimentation rate should be determined to screen for giant cell arteritis. The patient is then followed expectantly. If the neuropathy worsens or fails to improve by 3 months, then the patient should be further evaluated with a CT scan (with views of the base of the skull) and lumbar puncture.

Patients younger than 50 years (who are not diabetic or hypertensive) are not in the typical vasculopathic group and have a higher risk of underlying structural disease (e. g. , tumor). These patients should have a CT scan and lumbar puncture as part of their initial evaluation. An erythrocyte sedimentation rate and antinuclear antibody titer may additionally be of value to screen for an underlying vasculitis.

The pediatric patient with an isolated abducens nerve palsy should have a careful ostoscopic examination to detect otitis media and sinus films to rule out sinusitis. Abducens palsy may occur on a parainfectious basis following viral infection; a complete blood count with differential may be of value in detecting signs of preceding viral infection. These patients should be followed expectantly. The neuropathy usually resolves spontaneously over 6-12 weeks. If signs of progression or other neurologic deficits occur, then a more aggressive approach is indicated.

CAVERNOUS SINUS

The cavernous sinus is a paired parasellar venous structure which drains blood from the brain and the orbits. The oculomotor, trochlear, first and second divisions of trigeminal and abducens nerves pass through the cavernous sinus as they course from the brainstem to the orbit. Disease of the cavernous sinus, therefore, may result in dysfunction of these neural structures which lie in its wall. Several syndromes of the cavernous sinus which may present as emergencies are discussed.

Carotid-Cavernous Fistula

The syndrome of carotid-cavernous fistula results from an arterial communication with the cavernous sinus. There are two types of carotid-cavernous fistula. A connection from the internal carotid to the cavernous sinus can result in a direct high-flow fistula with the transmission of arterial pressure into a venous system. Connections between dural branches of the external carotid artery, alternatively, produces a low-flow "indirect" fistula.

The direct, high-flow type of carotid-cavernous fistula is more severe and may be complicated by visual loss. This type of fistula usually results from head trauma and may be associated with basilar skull fracture. External and internal ophthalmoplegias develop due to involvement of cranial nerves located in the wall of the cavernous sinus. Orbital venous congestion will cause proptosis and swelling. Congestion may compromise optic nerve perfusion and cause visual loss. The patient will typically complain of proptosis, ocular and periocular swelling, droopiness of the upper lid, binocular diplopia, and orbital pain. An audible intracranial "whooshing" sound may be noted by the patient as blood is diverted from the internal carotid into the cavernous sinus. Examination will reveal partial or complete external and internal ophthalmoplegia with moderate to severe orbital congestion. Proptosis, conjunctival injection and chemosis, arteriolization of conjunctival veins, and periocular swelling are usual findings. An elevated episcleral venous pressure usually causes an increased intraocular pressure. Fundus examination may reveal congested retinal veins. Auscultation of the orbit will usually reveal a bruit. Evaluation should include a CT scan with views to detect basilar skull fracture; carotid angiography will define the size and location of the fistula. Closure of the fistula via transarterial balloon catheter may be necessary to control pain and orbital congestion as well as to prevent irreversible visual loss.

The low-flow, indirect carotid-cavernous fistula is caused by connections with dural branches of the external carotid artery. This variant is much less severe and usually does not threaten to compromise vision. Unlike the high-flow type, the low-flow fistula usually occurs spontaneously. The patient will complain of ocular injection, irritation, and sometimes diplopia. Examination will reveal mild proptosis with conjunctival injection and arteriolization of conjunctival veins. Intraocular pressure is typically increased and fundus examination will reveal retinal vein fullness. Some degree of ophthalmoplegia may be noted depending upon the extent of cranial nerve involvement in the cavernous sinus. Auscultation of the orbit may reveal a bruit. These patients usually have a chronic course and are often seen for a chronic, unresponsive "conjunctivitis." The fistula often resolves spontaneously after weeks or months. If the symptoms from the fistula are particularly troublesome, or if the patient develops uncontrolled glaucoma, then more aggressive management may be necessary. Arteriography of the external carotids will reveal the site of the fistula and may also prove to be therapeutic (the fistula may close after angiography). Various embolization techniques have been used by neuroradiologists to close this type of fistula.

Cavernous Sinus Thrombosis

Cavernous sinus thrombosis is an uncommon but important cause of proptosis with ophthalmoplegia. Cavernous sinus thrombosis occurs as a result of transvenous spread of infection from one of the areas drained by the cavernous sinus (paranasal sinus, orbit, face, oropharynx). The cavernous sinus is a trabeculated structure with multiple channels which act as a "sieve." This property is thought to encourage the trapping of bacteria which subsequently leads to a septic thrombophlebitis. The patient may or may not give a history of preceding bacterial infection. Systemic symptoms include headache, shaking chills and fever, and generalized malaise. Again, orbital congestion is noted with chemosis, proptosis, periocular swelling, and a congestive retinopathy. Internal and external ophthalmoplegia may be noted secondary to cranial nerve involvement in the wall of the cavernous sinus. Hypesthesia in the distribution of the first and second divisions of the trigeminal nerve may also be noted. Signs of meningitis with an altered level of consciousness may be present. It is essential to recognize this entity early since prompt treatment with systemic antibiotics may prevent a fatal outcome. Prompt surgical drainage of the primary source of infection should be performed if necessary.

A thorough investigation should be initiated to locate the primary focus of infection if it is unclear on clinical examination; computerized tomography of the head and neck should be obtained to diagnose occult infection in the paranasal sinuses and pharynx.

Other Causes

Other causes of cavernous sinus disease which result in ophthalmoplegia include granulomatous inflammation (Tolosa-Hunt syndrome), various primary and metastatic tumors, intracavernous carotid aneurysm, and sphenoid mucocele. Evaluation always includes a CT scan of the sella and parasellar areas. Carotid angiography may be indicated to diagnose an aneurysm or to define tumor vascularity.

ORBIT

Patients with orbital disease may present with a variety of complaints and findings. Several important syndromes are described which may present as emergencies.

Graves' Disease

The ophthalmopathy of Graves' disease may cause a variety of symptoms. First and foremost, it is the most common cause of both unilateral and bilateral acquired proptosis. Other difficulties include pain, swelling, diplopia, and decreased vision. Symptoms often occur acutely and present as an ophthalmic emergency.

Patients with Graves' ophthalmopathy may be euthyroid, hypothyroid, or hyperthyroid. The onset of endocrine ophthalmopathy may be the harbinger of generalized thyrotoxicosis. There may be a past history of thyroid disease which is currently active or inactive. Typical symptoms of hyperthyroidism should be reviewed in cases of suspected Graves' ophthalmopathy. These include fever, weight loss, palpitations, nervousness, and heat intolerance.

Graves' ophthalmopathy is produced by an invasion of inflammatory cells into the orbit and extraocular muscles. Inflammation and edema of the orbital contents in the acute phase causes an orbital expansion with proptosis. Conjunctival injection results from both passive congestion and active inflammation. Levator involvement causes lid retraction. Swelling of the rectus muscles may result in restricted ductions. Posterior orbital involvement may cause an optic neuropathy. In the late fibrotic phase, fibroblasts predominate. Inflammatory signs improve but the normal tissue of the levator palpebrae and rectus muscles becomes replaced by scar tissue. Thus, restrictive myopathy and lid retraction tend to persist.

Findings on examination include unilateral or bilateral proptosis which is best followed quantitatively with an exophthalmometer. Other signs of ocular dysthyroidism may also be either unilateral or bilateral. Decreased visual acuity, impaired color vision, a Marcus-Gunn pupil, and visual field loss may be noted in cases complicated by optic neuropathy.

Resistance is usually encountered on attempted manual retropulsion of the globe through lightly closed lids. External examination (Fig. 11-10) may reveal lid and adnexal swelling. Conjunctival injection and edema are usually present and are often pronounced over the rectus muscle insertions. Lid retraction with exposure of the superior and inferior sclera may be noted in primary gaze ("thyroid stare"). Lid retraction may be so severe as to cause lagophthalmos; slit-lamp findings of

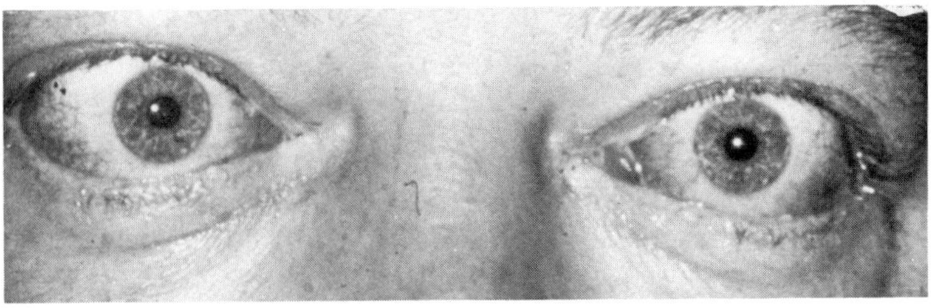

Fig. 11-10. Thyroid ophthalmopathy. (Courtesy, Wills Eye Hospital: Neuroophthalmology Unit).

exposure keratitis may be seen in these cases. "Lid lag" may be noted when the patient moves his eyes downward from upgaze; the upper eyelid "lags" behind that of the superior limbus. Misalignment of the globes in primary position may be noted; a hypertropia of the lesser-involved eye is most common. Ductional deficits may be noted in any field of gaze; deficient elevation is often seen because inferior rectus involvement is most frequent. Forced ductions, performed with a forceps or a cotton-tip applicator, will show that ductional changes are restrictive. Fundus examination may reveal disc swelling in cases complicated by optic neuropathy.

Laboratory studies of patients with suspected thyroid ophthalmopathy must include standard thyroid function tests. Computerized tomography of the orbits should be performed to document extraocular muscle swelling and to rule out the presence of retrobulbar tumor or mucocele. Confluence of swollen muscles on axial views may radiographically mimic a retrobulbar tumor; coronal cuts will best demonstrate muscle swelling and will prevent this misdiagnosis.

In the acute, inflammatory phase, a course of systemic steroids will make the patient more comfortable and reduce inflammation. Artificial tears and nightly application of ophthalmic ointment are helpful in cases with lagophthalmos. Systemic steroids are also indicated in patients with dysthyroid optic neuropathy. A persistent or progressive optic neuropathy which is unresponsive to steroids may require orbital irradiation or surgical decompression.

Orbital Pseudotumor

Orbital pseudotumor is an inflammatory disease which typically causes an acute or subacute painful proptosis with some degree of ophthalmoparesis. The pathophysiology involves focal or diffuse infiltration of nonspecific inflammatory tissue into any area of the orbit. All ages are affected and the process may be either bilateral or unilateral. Usual complaints include pain, swelling, proptosis, and diplopia. Pain is a more prominent feature in pseudotumor than with ocular dysthyroidism. Examination will typically reveal proptosis, lid edema, and conjunctival injection with chemosis. Involvement of the oculomotor or abducens nerves may produce ophthalmoparesis. Ductions may also be reduced secondary to restrictive myopathy (similar to Graves' disease) and proptosis. Patients with visual loss may be seen to have disc swelling or exudative retinal detachment (secondary to contiguous inflammation).

Evaluation must include CT scanning of the orbits and paranasal sinuses. Again, coronal views will better define the extraocular muscles. Rectus muscle swelling tends to involve the entire muscle diffusely (Fig. 11-11). In thyroid ophthalmopathy, the muscle belly is usually enlarged but tapers proximal to the insertion. No signs of bony destruction should be seen; bone erosion suggests a vasculitic or malignant process. Other studies to screen for an underlying vasculitis (e. g. , periarteritis nodosa) include an erythrocyte sedimentation rate, complete blood count, antinuclear antibody titer, and a urinalysis. A chest x-ray may be obtained to screen for lesions of Wegener's granulomatosis.

Treatment consists of high-dose oral prednisone. The patient will typically respond dramatically with rapid diminution of pain and inflammation. Steroids are then gradually tapered with careful observation for signs of exacerbation. Radiation therapy may also be considered for chronic cases, especially when complications include visual loss. Although some patients have a course of exacerbations and remissions, orbital pseudotumor tends to "burn out" and eventually become inactive. Recurrent or progressive disease requires orbital biopsy to rule out lymphoma; bone marrow biopsy may also be considered.

Orbital Cellulitis

Orbital cellulitis is a serious bacterial infection which may be rapidly progressive with potentially fatal complications.

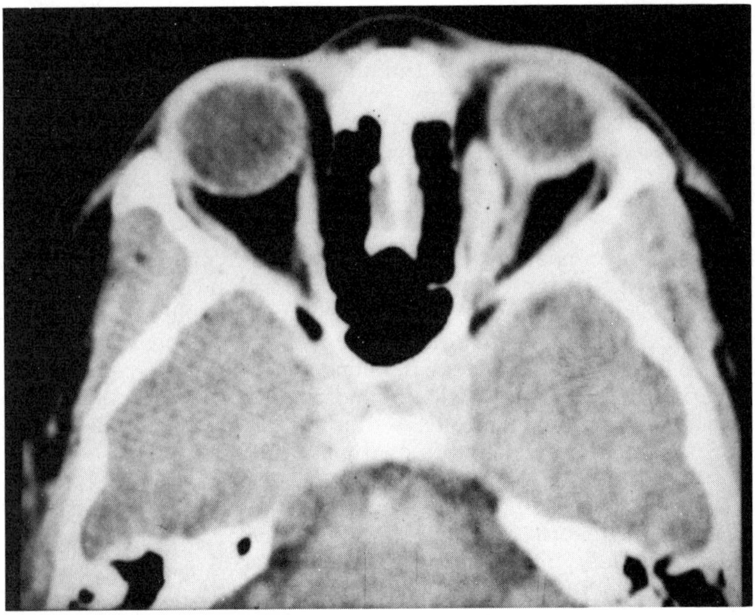

Fig. 11-11. Computerized tomography showing orbital myositis (pseudotumor).

Patients will complain of progressive orbital pain, swelling, and sometimes binocular diplopia. Systemic symptoms may include fever, chills, and malaise.

Findings on examination will include proptosis, lid swelling, conjunctival injection and chemosis, and orbital tenderness. Both neurogenic and restrictive ductional deficits may be noted. Upper lid ptosis and pupillary hyporeactivity suggest oculomotor nerve involvement. Disc swelling secondary to inflammation and orbital congestion is sometimes seen. Hypesthesia in the first division of the trigeminal nerve may be noted; involvement of the second division suggests cavernous sinus infection.

Laboratory findings usually include an elevated white blood count with a predominance of polymorphonuclear leukocytes and band cells. Blood and conjunctival cultures should be obtained; nasopharyngeal cultures may also be considered. Orbital cellulitis is frequently a complication of paranasal sinusitis. Studies must include a CT scan of the orbits with sinus views to rule out contiguous sinus infection. Changes suggestive of orbital abscess or osteomyelitis should also be noted. Finally, lumbar puncture should be performed in patients with suspected meningeal or cavernous sinus infection.

Treatment includes prompt administration of intravenous antibiotics. Gram-positive cocci and gram-negative rods are common infective agents. Initial coverage should include a penicillinase-resistant penicillin and an aminoglycoside (e. g. , methacillin and gentamicin). Young children must be covered with ampicillin or chloramphenicol for H. influenzae; the clinician should be aware of emerging ampicillin-resistant strains in some areas.

Antibiotics often produce dramatic improvement within 24 hours. Antibiotic therapy can be adjusted when culture results become available. Patients with sinusitis may require surgical drainage; early otorhinolaryngologic consultation will prepare for this possibility.

Diabetics and patients with other immunocompromising conditions require special consideration of mucormycosis (and other opportunistic infections) when orbital cellulitis develops. This rapidly progressive and usually fatal condition is potentially treatable when diagnosed early. The presence of ketoacidosis is thought to be a predisposing factor. Examination should include a search for necrotic nasal and oral lesions since the primary focus of infection is usually the nose, paranasal sinuses, or palate. The diagnosis is confirmed by prompt orbital, nasal, or oropharyngeal biopsy. Therapy consists of prompt surgical debridement with systemic antifungal therapy (e. g. , amphotericin B).

NEUROMUSCULAR JUNCTION

Myasthenia gravis (MG), the major cause of neuromuscular junction disease, is an autoimmune disorder which results from antibodies directed against the acetylcholine receptor at the muscle end plate. A disturbance in neuromuscular transmission results in the characteristic symptoms of muscle weakness and fatigability. MG may occur at any age but is most frequent in young females. A majority of patients present initially with ophthalmic complaints which include diplopia and upper lid ptosis. MG has two distinct syndromes: ocular and generalized myasthenia.

In ocular MG, signs and symptoms are limited to changes in ocular motility, lid position, and orbicularis weakness. About one-third of myasthenic patients will present with isolated ophthalmic symptoms. Approximately 50% of these patients will eventually develop generalized MG. After 2 years have passed, patients with isolated ocular MG are unlikely to develop generalized involvement. Initial complaints include upper lid ptosis and binocular diplopia. Symptoms often wax and wane, worsen with fatigue, and tend to be more pronounced at the end of the day. Examination may reveal upper lid ptosis with fatigability on prolonged upgaze. Manual elevation of the ptotic lid often causes the other lid to droop, producing "enhanced ptosis" (the "curtain" sign). After sustained downgaze, an upward vertical eye movement back to primary gaze may produce "Cogan's lid twitch." Orbicularis weakness is often seen on forced closure of the eyelids against manual resistance. MG may produce virtually any pattern of external ophthalmoparesis, with ductional deficits ranging from mild to severe. Motility changes often mimic neuropathic disorders, such as abducens palsy or INO (Fig. 11-12). The pupil is never affected clinically. A general neurologic examination should be performed to rule out generalized involvement.

Generalized MG, on the other hand, produces signs and symptoms of muscle weakness which include but are not limited to the ocular muscles. As was noted, one-half of the patients that present with isolated ocular MG initially will eventually convert to the generalized form. The patient with generalized MG will often complain of weakness and fatigue. Involvement of the bulbar musculature may lead to nasalized speech and dysphagia. Examination should focus on proximal muscle strength and fatigability.

The evaluation of suspected MG begins with the performance of a "tensilon test" using intravenous edraphonium. Edraphonium is a short-acting anticholinesterase which increases the quantity of acetylcholine at the neuromuscular junction. This will tend to reverse myasthenic weakness by saturating acetylcholine receptors with increased neurotransmitter. The tensilon test is best performed when there is a frank neurologic deficit (ptosis, motility disturbance) which can be easily assessed. To perform this procedure, 10 mg of edraphonium (total volume

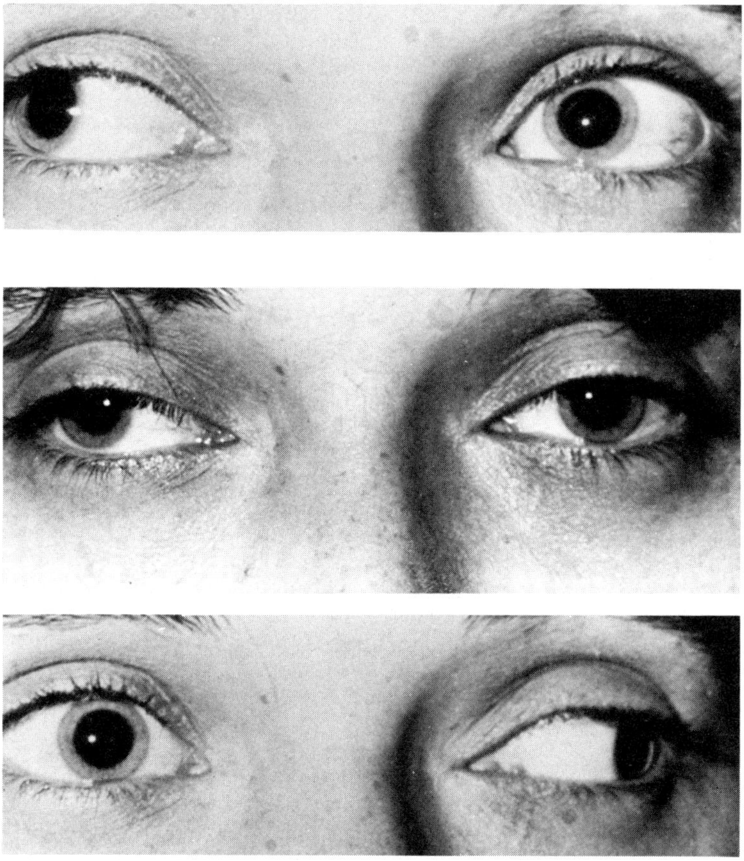

Fig. 11-12. Myasthenic pseudointernuclear ophthalmoplegia. (Courtesy, Wills Eye Hospital: Neuroophthalmology Unit).

1. 0 cc) is drawn up into a tuberculin syringe. The pretest neurologic deficit is then carefully observed as a baseline. Two mg (0. 2 cc) is then administered intravenously as a "test dose." If the deficit improves or resolves within 60 seconds, then the test is positive and the needle is removed. If the deficit remains unchanged, then the remainder of the edraphonium in the syringe is administered in 2-mg doses every 20 seconds until either improvement of the deficit or cholinergic symptoms (cramping, nausea) are noted. Atropine should be available to treat cholinergic side effects. Patients with cardiovascular disease should be monitored carefully.

The patient's evaluation should also include an assay for anti-acetylcholine receptor antibody. Due to an increased incidence of thymoma, a CT scan of the anterior mediastinum should be obtained. Neurologic consultation, of course, is indicated in any patient suspected of having myasthenia.

Anticholinesterase drugs and systemic steroids are the cornerstones of therapy. Anticholinesterases can be safely started on an outpatient basis. Pyridostigmine is started in doses of 30-60 mg orally every 8 hours and may be increased until myasthenic symptoms are relieved or the patient develops cholinergic side effects. Anticholinesterase drugs control ocular symptoms in only a minority of patients; oral steroids are more effective. Anticholinesterases should be the initial line of therapy, however, due to the incidence and severity of steroid-associated side effects. Initiation of steroid therapy, moreover, can cause a paradoxical rapid progression of weakness in generalized MG before antimyasthenic effects are obtained. For this reason, steroids should be started only on inpatients or under the close scrutiny of an experienced neurologist. Prednisone is then gradually tapered, with myasthenic symptoms being controlled often with comparatively low doses. Other forms of therapy for difficult cases of generalized MG include thymectomy, immunosuppression with azathioprine, and plasmapharasis.

SPECIAL TOPICS

TRANSIENT VISUAL LOSS

The evaluation of transient visual loss must start with an orderly and accurate history. The onset, severity, and duration of visual symptoms must be reviewed in detail. Any prodromal symptoms should be noted. The character of visual loss must be carefully explored with the crucial issue being whether one or both eyes are affected. The pattern of visual field loss may be important since patients may experience altitudinal or hemianopic defects. The frequency of visual disturbances should be determined; of particular importance are symptoms which are progressing in frequency, duration, and severity. Finally, the presence of accompanying neurologic or cardiovascular symptoms (e. g. , hemiparesis or diplopia) should be detailed.

Monocular Transient Visual Loss

Amaurosis fugax is the most important cause of transient monocular visual loss. Typically, the patient will describe a visual disturbance in which a "curtain" moves vertically across the visual field (either from above or below) and vision becomes "smoky." Visual loss may be only partial or may even progress to no light perception (NLP). Vision typically will return in a reverse fashion over 2-5 minutes; visual loss may occasionally persist for several hours.

Amaurosis fugax usually results from an embolic shower to the retinal circulation, most frequently arising from an atheromatous carotid bifurcation. Less commonly, emboli may be of cardiac origin; underlying causes include valvular disease, atrial fibrillation, and mural thrombus. Amaurosis fugax may also precede an arteritic ischemic optic neuropathy secondary to giant cell arteritis.

Evaluation of the patient with amaurosis fugax should include carotid and cardiac auscultation, measurement of blood pressure, and a fundus examination to rule out embolic plaques. Cholesterol emboli are yellow and refractile (Hollenhorst plaques); platelet aggregates are often white and creamy in appearance. Patients with amaurosis fugax should be referred to a neurologist for evaluation and treatment. Tests available for evaluation of suspected carotid disease include ultrasonography, doppler studies, oculoplethysmography, digital subtraction angiography via intravenous contrast injection, and intraarterial angiography. The goal of carotid testing is to detect the presence of a hemodynamically significant stenotic lesion which may predispose to stroke. Echocardiography is indicated in cases of suspected valvular disease or mural thrombus; electrocardiography will document atrial fibrillation.

The management of amaurosis fugax is a controversial topic in neurology. Medical therapy consists of antiplatelet and anticoagulant drugs including aspirin, dipyridamole, warfarin, and heparin. Patients with stable amaurosis often enjoy complete symptomatic control on aspirin at a dose of 10 grains daily. Patients with the recent onset of amaurosis or those who fail on medical therapy may require more aggressive therapy. Carotid endarterectomy should be considered when significant degrees of carotid stenosis are found. Surgery may prevent the complications of impaired carotid blood flow which include cerebrovascular accident and ocular ischemia. The decision for carotid endarterectomy is sometimes difficult and must be made by the consulting neurologist. Factors which should be considered include the underlying diagnosis, the results of previous forms of treatment, the patient's age and medical condition, and the local morbidity rate for carotid surgery.

Certain patients with amaurosis fugax need particularly aggressive management. "Crescendo amaurosis" occurs when episodes of visual loss become progressively more severe with an increasing frequency and duration. Patients with demonstrable residual deficits (e. g. , branch retinal artery occlusion) also need very prompt evaluation. These patients may require hospital admission with heparinization to prevent impending stroke or central retinal artery occlusion. After the amaurosis has been stabilized, then the evaluation as to underlying etiology may proceed so that appropriate management can be undertaken.

Other less common causes of transient monocular visual loss should also be considered. Giant cell arteritis may present with amaurosis fugax which foreshadows an arteritic ischemic optic neuropathy; the evaluation of elderly patients with amaurosis fugax should include an erythrocyte sedimentation rate. Patients with papilledema may experience transient visual obscurations which last several seconds; these episodes are considerably briefer than true amaurosis and are provoked by postural changes. Examination of the discs will reveal swelling typical of papilledema. Retinal migraine may cause monocular visual loss lasting less than 10 minutes; the patient will usually have a history of previous migraine-type phenomena. Other conditions which occasionally present with transient visual loss include disc drusen and myopia.

Binocular Transient Visual Loss

The finding of monocular visual changes localizes pathophysiology to the optic nerve or globe; binocular visual loss, on the other hand, implies chiasmal or retrochiasmal disease. Transient binocular visual loss often results from ischemia involving the occipital cortex or optic radiations. Cerebrovascular disease and migraine are the two most important causes of binocular visual disturbances.

Vertebrobasilar insufficiency may cause transient occipital lobe ischemia; homonymous hemianopic visual disturbances lasting minutes to hours may result. Bilateral occipital involvement may produce a complete binocular "gray-out" of vision. A careful history must be taken regarding the pattern of visual loss. Patients tend to lateralize symptoms toward the eye with the temporal field deficit (e. g. , a patient with a transient right homonymous hemianopia may actually complain of a visual disturbance in the right eye). The patient should be asked whether he covered each eye separately to test for binocularity of symptoms. Other symptoms of brainstem dysfunction which may accompany the visual disturbance include diplopia (e. g. , skew deviation, INO), oscillopsia (nystagmus), nausea, vertigo, dysphagia, dysarthria, and hemiparesis.

Evaluation of patients with suspected vertebrobasilar insufficiency includes measuring the blood pressure in both arms and formal perimetry to outline any residual visual field defect. A prompt neurology referral is needed for thorough evaluation and to plan therapy.

Amaurosis fugax (monocular visual loss) is the typical visual disturbance produced by anterior circulation ischemia. Hemispheric ischemia usually presents as a neurologic emergency with transient ischemic attack (TIA). Even though involvement of the optic radiations may cause a transient homonymous hemianopia, complaints of hemiparesis or hemisensory disturbance usually predominate at the time of presentation.

Other causes of transient binocular visual loss should be considered. Migraine (discussed in the next section) commonly has an associated homonymous visual disturbance. A fluctuating blood glucose in uncontrolled diabetes can cause osmotic lens changes with a varying myopia (and a bilateral visual disturbance). Occipital lobe arteriovenous malformations and neoplasms may sometimes cause visual hallucinations with flashing lights and jagged lines which mimic migraine phenomena. The patient with multiple migraine attacks which always involve the same side of the visual field should have a CT scan to rule out a structural lesion.

MIGRAINE

Migraine disorders are characterized by the occurrence of episodic headache which is accompanied by vascular changes in the intracranial and extracranial arterial circulations. Patients with migraine frequently present to the emergency room as ophthalmologic emergencies. Associated ophthalmic symptoms may include homonymous binocular visual disturbances, transient monocular visual loss, and photophobia. Nausea and vomiting frequently accompany migraine headaches. Migraine disorders usually begin in chillhood or early adult life and tend to diminish in middle age; migraine may, however, reappear in the elderly. A history of motion sickness during childhood and a family history of migraine headaches are commonly present. Varieties of migraine include common, classic, complicated, basilar, retinal, and ophthalmoplegic migraine.

Common migraine presents with a severe headache which initially starts with throbbing hemicranial pain but then progresses into a dull, generalized headache which is accompanied by nausea. Headaches last for hours to days and frequently cause patients to seek out a quiet, darkened environment in which to recuperate. Eye symptoms may include ocular pain, conjunctival injection, tearing, periorbital swelling, and photophobia.

Classic migraine differs from the common variety in that it is preceded by a prodrome (aura) of characteristic visual changes or other neurologic symptoms. Visual changes often include bright lights (photopsia) with zig-zag lines (fortifications) which begin centrally in both eyes and then expand toward the periphery in a homonymous fashion. As the fortifications spread, they tend to leave a homonymous visual field defect (scotoma which the patient perceives as a "blind spot"). This scenario typically lasts 15 minutes and is followed by a typical common migraine headache. The aura can include other neurologic symptoms such as hemiparesis, hemisensory loss, or aphasia. Sometimes the aura is not followed by headache, thus simulating cerebrovascular disease. When this occurs in middle-aged or elderly patients, a careful history will often reveal previous migraine during early life.

Complicated migraine occurs when neurologic deficits persist beyond the normal 15-minute interval. Neurologic deficits may persist for hours, days, or may even be permanent.

Basilar migraine refers to migraine headaches which are preceded by deficits in the basilar artery distribution. These may include occipital visual loss, ataxia, diplopia, dysarthria, vertigo, and even loss of consciousness. This disorder is distinguished from ischemic vascular disease by the presence of the typical migraine headache, a past history of similar recurrent episodes without residual deficit, and the young age of the patient.

Retinal migraine is a rare disorder producing transient monocular visual loss lasting about 10 minutes; the visual disturbance does not include a scintillating scotoma and often is not followed by headache. Recurrent episodes may lead to a permanent residual visual deficit. This diagnosis is facilitated when the visual deficit is accompanied by a typical migraine headache; otherwise, this is largely a diagnosis of exclusion after other causes of monocular visual loss have been ruled out.

Ophthalmoplegic migraine is a rare disorder which always begins by age 10 and is characterized by ophthalmoplegia which follows a typical migraine headache. Oculomotor palsy is the most common etiology of the motility disturbance. Although ophthalmoplegia usually resolves spontaneously, it may become chronic after the occurrence of repeated episodes.

Cluster headache is a related disorder which is usually seen in young adult males. This patient typically complains of severe unilateral facial pain which is associated with ipsilateral tearing, nasal congestion, and facial flushing. The headache usually lasts about 45 minutes. These episodes may occur daily for weeks to months (in a "clustered" pattern) followed by a symptom-free interval of weeks to months. Often there is an associated Horner's syndrome on the involved side which clears along with the other symptoms. The head pain is often severe and incapacitating; patients tend to walk around with their headache rather than lie in a quiet room. If neurologic deficits other than a Horner's syndrome occur, then an underlying lesion in the orbit or cavernous sinus should be considered.

The treatment of migraine disorders starts with controlling the acute headache; prophylaxis against further episodes is then undertaken. Patients with acute migraine headaches should be treated with analgesics as required. Propanolol is currently the drug of choice for prophylactic treatment of migraine phenomena. The usual starting dose is 10 mg 3 times a day; it is then increased as necessary until the episodes are controlled. Methysergide 1-2 mg 4 times a day is also an effective prophylactic medication; complications of retroperitoneal and pulmonary fibrosis have been noted after long-term use. Amitriptyline is another beneficial prophylactic medication; the usual starting dose of 25 mg at bedtime is increased as required to 75 mg daily. Patients with classic migraine may be treated with ergotomine preparations during the onset of the aura in order to prevent the subsequent headache. A 2-mg dose is taken sublingually, followed if necessary by 2 mg every 1 hour up to a total maximum dose of 6 mg.

NYSTAGMUS

Nystagmus is a to-and-fro oscillatory eye movement which often changes in character in different fields of gaze. The subjective correlate of nystagmus is oscillopsia, a phenomenon in which the patient perceives the environment to move back and forth in a rhythmic fashion. Nystagmus is categorized by the pattern of ocular oscillation. Horizontal and vertical nystagmus refer to the plane of eye movements. In pendular nystagmus, the eyes move with equal velocity in each direction; jerk nystagmus, on the other hand, has rapid and slow phases for each direction of the oscillation. Jerk nystagmus is named by the direction of the rapid phase; thus, nystagmus which has its quick phase toward the right is termed "right-beating" nystagmus. In torsional nystagmus, the eyes rotate in a rhythmic fashion. Other forms of nystagmus include circular, elliptical, and convergence retraction.

The most common neuroophthalmic emergency associated with nystagmus occurs when the patient presents to the emergency room with an acute onset of vertigo. The clinician is called upon to differentiate a relatively benign acute peripheral vestibular disorder (e. g. , acute labyrinthitis) from a potentially serious central disorder such as brainstem infarction. The presence of other neurologic findings produced by brainstem stroke (e. g. , dysarthria, diplopia, or hemiparesis) may facilitate the diagnosis of a central etiology. When these signs are absent, however, the pattern of nystagmus may help differentiate peripheral from central disease.

Unilateral peripheral vestibular disease (e. g. , labyrinthitis) produces a mixed horizontal and torsional nystagmus. The horizontal component is unidirectional; that is, the quick phase moves in the same direction regardless of whether the patient looks to the right or to the left. Nystagmus is most prominent when the eyes are deviated in the direction of the fast phase. Although the direction of the horizontal component does not change in contralateral gaze, it will typically have a smaller amplitude. In addition, peripheral vestibular disorders tend to produce more severe vertigo and nausea than brainstem disease.

Central vestibular disease (e. g. , brainstem infarction) usually produces bidirectional nystagmus; the horizontal component of the nystagmus is seen to be right-beating in the right gaze and left-beating in the left gaze. Purely vertical nystagmus may be seen. Vertigo is typically mild.

Other forms of nystagmus will rarely present as an emergency but may be noted when the patient presents with an unrelated problem. Congenital nystagmus is present from birth and is usually horizontal and pendular, even in upgaze. The nystagmus is often seen to have a reduced amplitude in one particular field of gaze, the so-called null point. The patient tends to spontaneously keep his head turned so that his nystagmus is minimal while looking straight ahead. The nystagmus is typically increased by attempted fixation and may be dampened by convergence. Latent nystagmus refers to an ocular oscillation which occurs when one eye is covered. This may be associated with esotropia and is always a benign condition. Convergence-retraction nystagmus is often seen with dorsal midbrain lesions. Bilateral ocular retraction and convergence occur on attempted upgaze. Associated findings are an impairment of upgaze, pupillary light-near dissociation and upper lid retraction. Downbeat nystagmus may be seen with disease of the craniocervical junction. This is a vertical nystagmus with the fast component directed downward and is accentuated on downgaze. Downbeat nystagmus is always pathologic and requires further neurologic evaluation.

ANISOCORIA

Anisocoria refers to an inequality of the pupils. Anisocoria is either physiologic or due to disease of the efferent system; afferent disorders never result in pupillary inequality. Sympathetic pathways innervate the iris dilator muscles while parasympathetic nerves supply the iris sphincter muscle (via the oculomotor nerve). Inequality may be produced by assymmetric disease affecting one of these two systems. Unilateral disease of the iris (e. g. , postinflammatory damage of sphincter tear) may also produce anisocoria. Finally, exposure to topical agents may produce "atropinic" dilation of one eye. When these other disorders have been excluded, the diagnosis of simple (physiologic) anisocoria is made.

Fig. 11-13 shows a scheme by which the clinician can logically evaluate anisocoria. The first step involves checking the light reaction and comparing pupillary size when examined in both bright and dim illumination. A good light reaction implies that

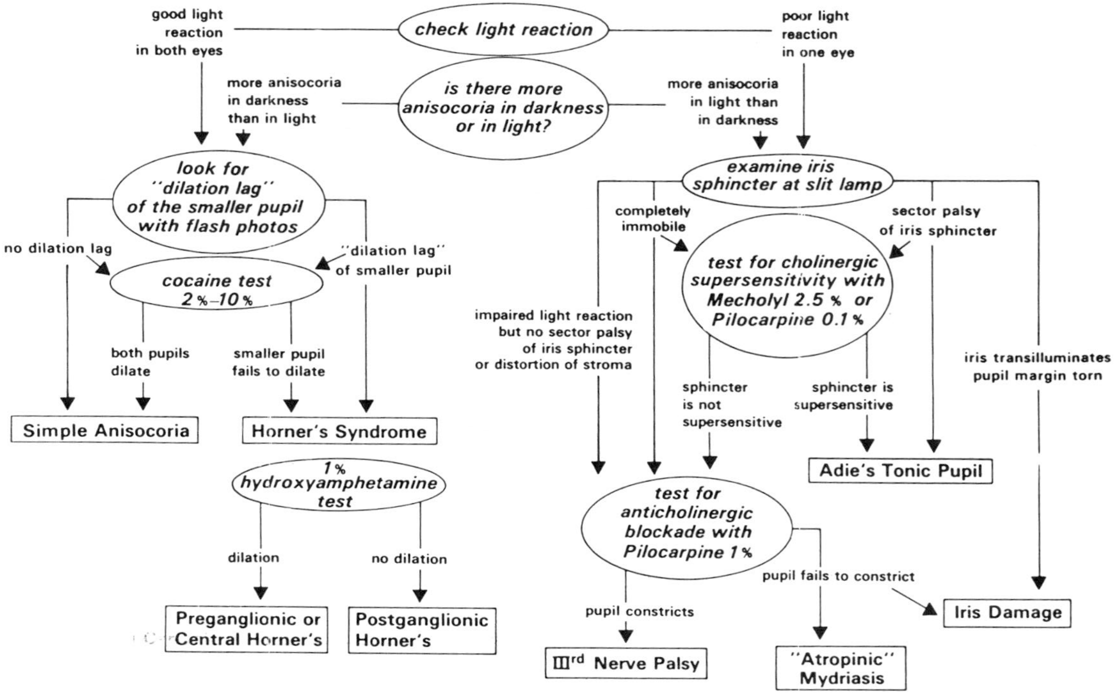

Fig. 11-13. Flow chart for evaluation of anisocoria. (Reproduced, with permission, from Thompson, H.S. and Pilley, S.F.J.: Unequal pupils. A flow chart for sorting out the anisocorias. Surv Ophth 21(1):46, 1976.)

the innervation of the pupillary sphincter is normal. When anisocoria is greater in the dark, the iris dilator muscle may be weakened suggesting a sympathetic lesion. Examination with a slit lamp may reveal signs of iris atrophy or a tear of the pupillary sphincter muscle. Pharmacologic testing of the pupil can further be performed to aid in the diagnosis of anisocoria. Topical cocaine and hydroxyamphetamine are used to sort out lesions of the sympathetic system while topical pilocarpine may aid in the evaluation of the parasympathetic system.

A Horner's syndrome is produced by a sympathetic pathway lesion. The involved eye typically has a miotic pupil with anisocoria being greater in the dark than under bright illumination. Two or three millimeters of upper lid ptosis is a usual finding due to the involvement of Muller's muscle. Topical 10% cocaine may be applied to confirm the presence of Horner's pupil; the normal pupil will become mydriatic while the miotic pupil will fail to dilate.

Preganglionic lesions of the sympathetic pathways occur proximal to the superior cervical ganglion. Unilateral facial anhydrosis is usually seen with preganglionic lesions due to involvement of sweat fibers which are distributed with the external carotid artery. An important cause of a preganglionic Horner's syndrome is the Pancoast tumor which involves sympathetic fibers as they course over the lung. Postganglionic sympathetic lesions are produced by sympathetic pathway involvement distal to the superior cervical ganglion. The Horner's syndrome of cluster headaches is characteristically postganglionic. Topical 1% hydroxyamphetamine is used to differentiate preganglionic from postganglionic lesions; this medication will cause the preganglionic pupil to dilate while the postganglionic pupil will fail to dilate.

Slit-lamp examination may reveal signs of previous iris injury which results in mydriasis and pupillary hyporeactivity. A previous episode of iritis may have produced iris atrophy, while old trauma may have caused a tear in the pupillary sphincter.

Adie's tonic pupil is produced by a lesion of the parasympathetic pathways. The pupil is typically mydriatic and is seen to have light-near dissociation; that is, there is a poor reaction to light stimulation but the pupil does become more miotic during attempted near fixation. Vermiform (worm-like) movements of the pupil may be noted on slit-lamp examination. This condition is produced by lesions involving the ciliary ganglion (e.g., herpes zoster). A phenomenon known as denervation hypersensitivity develops and the iris becomes very sensitive to topical parasympathomimetic agents. This may be confirmed by application of topical 0.12% pilocarpine. The hypersensitive Adie's pupil will constrict while the normal pupil will not appreciably change. This is a benign condition which requires no further evaluation.

Oculomotor palsy will produce anisocoria when parasympathetic fibers innervating the pupillary sphincter muscle are involved. Mydriasis and hyporeactivity of the involved pupil will be seen. Associated findings include ptosis of the upper eyelid (due to levator palpebrae weakness) and ophthalmoparesis (due to superior, medial, and inferior rectus weakness). As previously discussed, an acute pupil-involving oculomotor palsy constitutes a neurosurgical emergency when caused by a compressive posterior communicating artery aneurysm. When associated lid and motility findings are absent, pharmacologic testing with topical 1% pilocarpine may help differentiate parasympathoparesis from a pharmacologically dilated pupil as outlined below.

The pharmacologically dilated pupil is typically widely dilated and completely unreactive. This may be seen among medical personnel who inadvertently or intentionally instill an anticholinergic agent (e.g., atropine) into one eye. This suspected diagnosis may be confirmed with topical 1% pilocarpine. The pharmacologically dilated pupil will fail to constrict after application of this agent while the pupil with a true parasympathoparesis will constrict to some degree.

BIBLIOGRAPHY

Adams, R.D. and Victor, M.: Principles of Neurology, 2nd ed. McGraw-Hill, New York, 1981.

Asbury, A.K., Aldridge, H., Hershberg, R., et al.: Oculomotor palsy in diabetes mellitus. Brain 93:555-556, 1970.

Boghen, D.R. and Glaser, J.S.: Ischemic optic neuropathy. The clinical profile and natural history. Brain 98:689-708, 1975.

Cogan, D.G.: Neurology of the Ocular Muscles, 2nd ed. Charles C Thomas, Springfield, IL, 1956.

Cogan, D.G. and Williams, H.W.: Neurology of the Visual System. Charles C Thomas, Springfield, IL, 1966.

Glaser, J.D.: Neuro-Ophthalmology. Harper and Row, Hagerstown, MD, 1978.

Goodman, B.W.: Temporal arteritis. Am J Med 67:839-852, 1979.

Jakobiec, F.A. and Jones, I.S.: Orbital inflammations. In Duane, T.D. (ed.): Clinical Ophthalmology, vol. 2. Harper and Row, Hagerstown, MD, 1980.

Miller, N.R.: Myasthenia gravis: Systemic and ocular considerations. Ophthalmology 86:2165-2174, 1979.

Rosenberg, M.A., Savino, P.J., and Glaser, J.S.: A clinical analysis of pseudopapilledema. I. Population, laterality, acuity, refractive error, ophthalmoscopic characteristics, and coincident disease. Arch Ophth 97:65-70, 1979.

Savino, P.J., Glaser, J.S., and Rosenberg, M.A.: A clinical analysis of pseudopapilledema. II. Visual field defects. Arch Ophth 97:71-75, 1979.

Scheie, H.G. and Albert, D.M.: Adler's Textbook of Ophthalmology. W.B. Saunders, Philadelphia, 1969.

Sergott, R.C. and Glaser, J.S.: Graves' ophthalmopathy: A clinical and immunological review. Surv Ophth 26:1-21, 1981.

Thompson, H.S. and Pilley, S.F.J.: Unequal pupils. A flow chart for sorting out the anisocorias. Surv Ophth 21:45-48, 1976.

Trobe, J.D., Glaser, J.S., and LaFlamme, P.: Dysthyroid optic neuropathy. Clinical profile and rationale for management. Arch Ophth 96:1199-1209, 1978.

Walsh, F.B. and Hoyt, W.F.: Clinical Neuro-Ophthalmology, 3rd ed. Williams and Wilkins, Baltimore, 1969.

Chapter 12

PEDIATRIC OPHTHALMOLOGIC EMERGENCIES

Children are subject to the same types of ocular injuries as adults. There is an increased frequency of eye trauma secondary to projectile injury in the pediatric age group. Since one cannot anticipate a great deal of cooperation from a frightened child, a systematic, methodical exam is essential. Emphasis must be placed on techniques that maximize the information obtained with minimal intervention.

HISTORY

The history of the injury or ocular complaint is taken from the child, when able, and from the parents or other witnesses. Just as in adults, chemical injuries should be treated immediately with copious irrigation with water or saline.

Once the nature of the injury has been determined, additional pertinent information is elicited. It is important to know when the child last ate, should surgery be necessary. Of course the child must be evaluated for other injuries. Extensive facial trauma, bilateral corneal abrasions, unexplained hyphemas, retinal hemorrhages, and cigarette burns should raise the possibility of a battered child. If this is considered, pediatric consultation is essential.

The history directs the examiner toward a particular diagnostic evaluation. A past history of ocular disease, trauma, or poor vision as with amblyopia may be important if the visual loss or extent of injury is inconsistent with the history. A prior history of strabismus may be significant. Naturally, a history of systemic disease in the child may help in explaining the ocular findings.

EXAMINATION

VISUAL ACUITY

Depending on the nature of the injury (abrasion or foreign body), irritation may be so extensive, that a topical anesthetic may be necessary to examine the eye, even to record a visual acuity. One drop of either tetracaine hydrochloride or proparacaine hydrochloride will provide adequate anesthesia. Vision is best evaluated with a Snellen letter chart, isolated E, or picture chart. Pocket screeners for near acuity are helpful if a distance acuity chart (20 feet or 6 meters) is unavailable. It is essential to record the visual acuity measured both with and without correction if the child wears glasses. An attempt to improve the acuity with a pinhole should be made.

In the preverbal or anxious child, the ability to fixate on and follow an interesting object or light with one eye occluded is recorded. The examiner can use a piece of tape or his hand to occlude one eye while he observes the other (Fig. 12-1). If the child resists occlusion of one eye more than the other, poorer vision is suspected in the opposite nonoccluded eye. The vision is recorded as "fixes and follows light or a measured object or does not follow light," etc. Frequently one can only determine that a child reacts to a bright light by avoidance, and light perception (LP) is recorded as the vision. Again, a great deal of information is obtained by observing changes in the child's behavior when one or the other eye is occluded. In these cases poor vision can be suspected, particularly if there is evidence of unilateral ocular disease or injury.

EXAMINATION TECHNIQUES

If the child is cooperative, a stepwise evaluation as delineated in the chapter on Eye Examination is carried out. This chapter is directed to the infant and preverbal child unwilling or unable to cooperate.

An external examination of the skin, lids, and adnexae can be

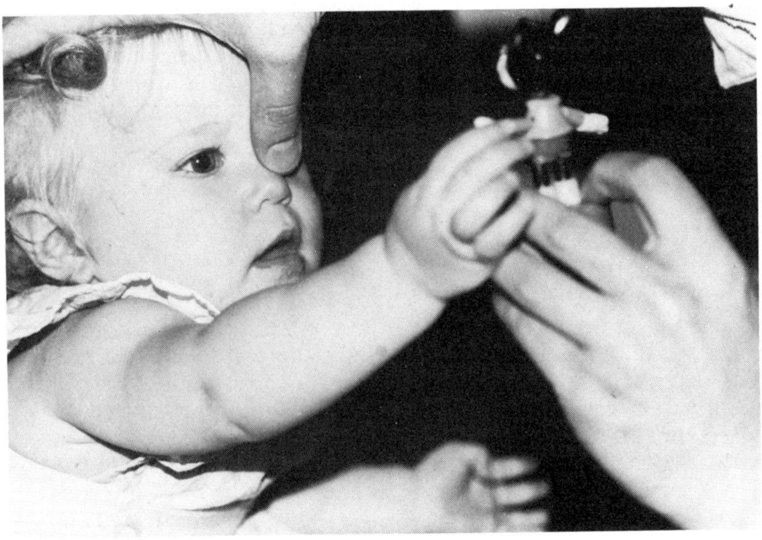

Fig. 12-1. Examiner occludes left eye with thumb and observes child's fixation on toy.

easily performed by inspection in good lighting, with minimal contact. It is preferable for the parent to hold the child during the exam to decrease anxiety. A papoose type restraint may be needed particularly if lid suturing is required.

To examine the eye and palpebral conjunctiva instillation of a topical anesthetic may be helpful. A light source is essential (pen light) and magnification helpful. Forceful eye lid opening when necessary can be accomplished with a lid speculum (Fig. 12-2). Cotton swabs held close to the lid margin and rolled to open the lids work very well (Fig. 12-3).

Once the lids are opened, careful inspection of the eye is begun. As in the adult the conjunctiva and cornea are inspected and sterile fluorescein solution instilled if indicated. Use of a Wood's lamp will easily demonstrate an abrasion of the cornea. The pupil is examined for reactivity and irregularity of shape which may be indicative of a ruptured globe. Other signs of perforation, such as shallow anterior chamber and prolapse of uveal tissue, are noted. Recognition of a hyphema is important, since these children are usually hospitalized as part of their treatment.

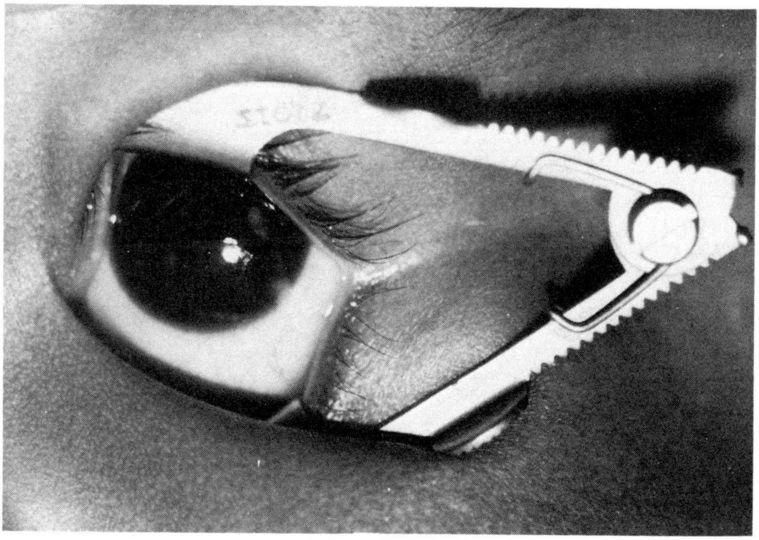

Fig. 12-2. Lid speculum used to open eye for examination after instillation of topical anesthetic.

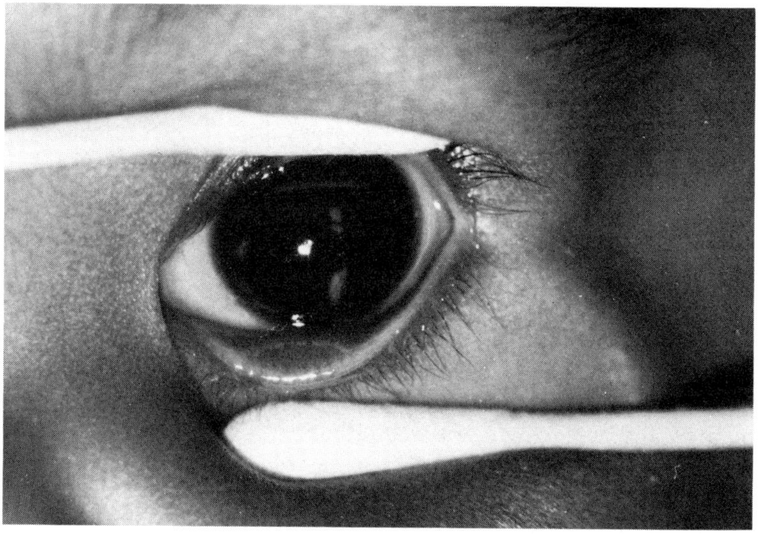

Fig. 12-3. Cotton applicators used to open eyelids.

Should conjunctivitis or cellulitis be suspected, appropriate scrapings and cultures are taken prior to instituting specific antibiotic therapy. An attempt to observe a red fundus reflex with a direct ophthalmoscope at +10 held 12 inches from the patient is made. This will help to diagnose media opacities, such as cataracts and intraocular tumors.

A retinal exam is then performed, using the direct or indirect ophthalmoscope if available. Hand-held slit lamps are available which make the evaluation of the child's eye easier, for example, in diagnosing anterior uveitis (Fig. 12-4).

SPECIFIC PEDIATRIC EMERGENCIES

In general, the treatment of most pediatric eye emergencies is the same as for the adult. Specific types of injuries and their treatments are discussed in the appropriate chapters in this book. There are, however, a few conditions which present almost exclusively in the pediatric age group, for which immediate recognition and treatment is essential.

CONGENITAL GLAUCOMA

This is characterized by an increase in intraocular pressure leading to ocular damage and visual loss in early childhood. It is believed to be the result of a genetically determined defect in the filtration angle in the anterior chamber of the eye. Presenting signs include epiphora, photophobia, blepharospasm, and corneal haze and enlargement. Of course, cupping of the optic nerve head occurs secondarily. These children characteristically present in the first year of life, often before 6 months of age.

Corneal haze secondary to edema is the finding that most often brings the infant to medical attention, frequently to the emergency room (Fig. 12-5). The suspicion or recognition of this condition must be followed by immediate ophthalmologic referral. The treatment of congenital glaucoma is surgical either by a goniotomy or by a trabeculotomy.

LEUKOKORIA (WHITE PUPILLARY REFLEX)

A white pupil may have been noticed by the parents either in photographs or when the child's gaze is directed a certain way (Fig. 12-6). The examiner may notice it when attempting to

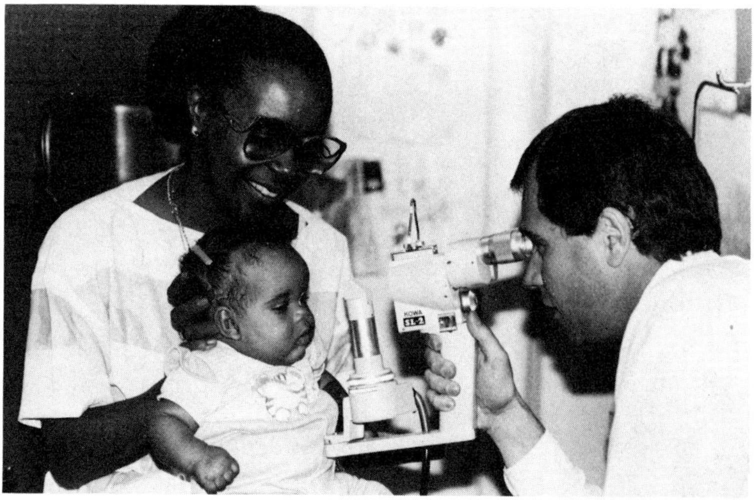

Fig. 12-4. Hand-held slit lamp used for anterior segment examination.

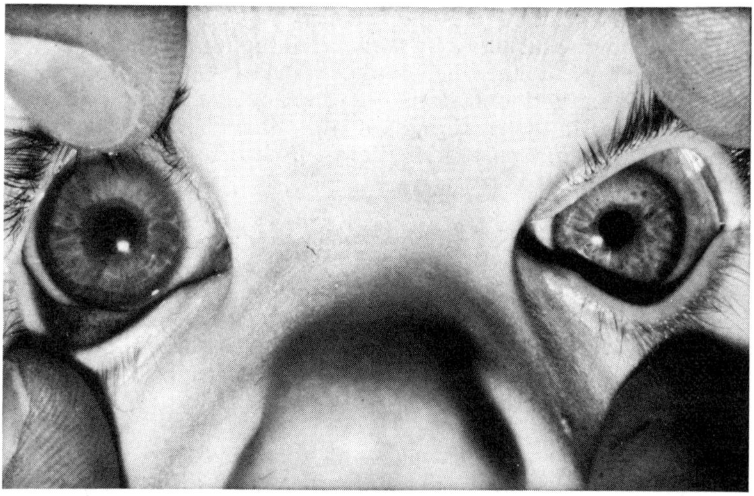

Fig. 12-5. Infant with congenital glaucoma and corneal enlargement of the right eye.

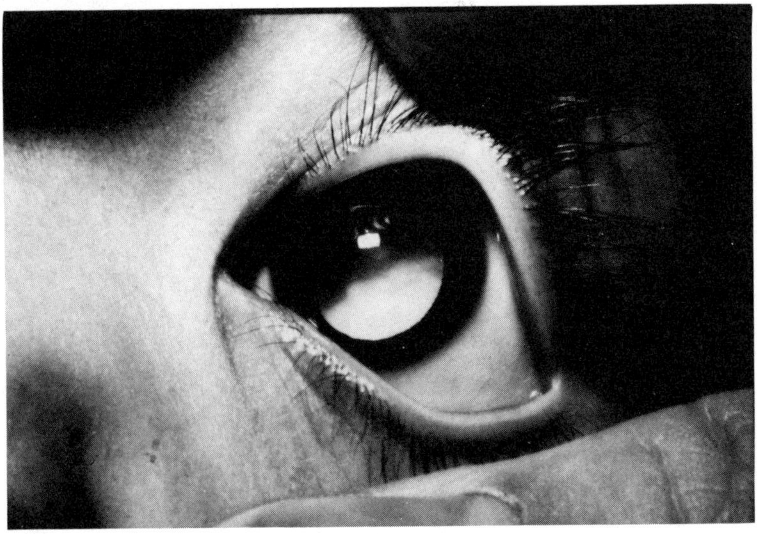

Fig. 12-6. Leukokoria in child with retinoblastoma.

visualize the red fundus reflex or retina with the direct ophthalmoscope. This finding may be secondary to a number of conditions including cataracts, intraocular infection, intraocular tumor, and retrolental fibroplasia. Certainly the most ominous cause is a retinoblastoma, an intraocular tumor, which often presents in the first year of life either unilaterally or bilaterally. At any rate immediate referral is mandatory when leukokoria is found.

ACUTE ONSET OF STRABISMUS

Any child presenting with an acute onset of strabismus should have a complete neurologic exam. Although a decompensated phoria may suddenly present as a constant manifest deviation, as in a hyperope with an accommodative esotropia, neurologic causes must be excluded.

Sixth nerve palsies presenting as an esotropia may occur following a viral illness, but may also be a sign of increased intracranial pressure. A hypertropia following closed heat trauma may be secondary to a fourth nerve palsy. Oculomotor nerve palsies may be a sign of ophthalmologic migraine but may also be secondary to an aneurysm as in the adult age group. The diagnosis and treatment of these conditions is discussed in Chapter 11.

OCULAR MANIFESTATIONS OF CHILD ABUSE

Approximately 40% of children with the battered-child syndrome have associated ocular findings. Intraocular hemorrhage often associated with intracranial bleeding is the most common ocular finding. Periorbital swelling and ecchymosis, hyphemas, cataracts, and dislocated lenses may be secondary to this type of trauma. The examiner should be suspicious of child abuse whenever an eye injury cannot be explained adequately. Fractures and soft-tissue injuries in various stages of healing and cigarette burns to the skin may help to confirm the diagnosis. Appropriate referral is mandatory for these unfortunate children.

BIBLIOGRAPHY

Frey, T.: Pediatric eye trauma. Pediatric Annals 12:487-497, 1983.

Friendly, D. S.: Ocular manifestations of physical child abuse. Trans Amer Acad Ophthal Otolaryngol 75:318, 1971.

Harley, R. D.: Pediatric Ophthalmology, 2nd ed. W. B. Saunders, Philadelphia, 1983.

Nelson, L. B.: Symposium on Pediatric Ophthalmology. The Pediatric Clinics of North America. Vol. 30 No. 6, December 1983. W. B. Saunders, Philadelphia.

Shields, J. A.: Diagnosis and Management of Intraocular Tumors. Chapter 17, in Differential Diagnosis of Retinoblastoma, pp. 497-533. C. V. Mosby Co., St. Louis, 1983.

APPENDIX I: EVALUATION OF OCULAR COMPLAINTS OR SYMPTOMS

At times a person may present with no specific complaint and would like to have a routine examination. However, most people do present with a chief complaint and associated symptoms. It is the interpretation and evaluation of these complaints that leads to the proper diagnosis and treatment. This appendix presents the evaluation of what is suggested or what has possibly occurred in regard to the specific complaints.

COMPLAINTS WITH A VISUAL COMPONENT

SUDDEN LOSS OF VISION IN ONE EYE

This is a more common complaint than sudden loss of vision in both eyes. Occlusion of the central retinal artery or vein, total retinal detachment and massive vitreous or retinal hemorrhages are easily diagnosed with an ophthalmoscope. Other conditions causing this problem, i. e. , optic neuritis (papillitis or retrobulbar), internal carotid artery occlusion, toxic amblyopia, and skull injury with edema, hemorrhage, or fracture of the optic foramen, require a more extensive evaluation.

SUDDEN LOSS OF VISION IN BOTH EYES

This is a rarer complaint and should lead one to think of the following: extensive head injury, toxic amblyopia (tobacco, chloroquine, methyl alcohol), optic neuritis, migraine, malingering, or hysteria.

GRADUAL LOSS OF VISION IN ONE OR BOTH EYES

This is a much more common complaint than either of the two sudden losses of vision. This complaint may be the result of an uncorrected refractive error or a pathological condition. These two causes may be differentiated with the use of a pinhole. If the visual acuity improves with the pinhole, the cause is at least partially, a refractive error. If the visual acuity does not improve or worsens with the pinhole the cause is pathological.

Refractive error may be myopia, hyperopia, astigmatism or presbyopia, changes in diabetes secondary to uncontrolled blood sugar levels, early keratoconus, lens sclerosis, lens subluxation, elevated macula or retina secondary to a retrobulbar mass, ocular tumor, serous retinopathy, or lid pressure secondary to lid inflammation, edema, or ptosis.

Pathological conditions can involve any of the ocular structures which may interfere with the visual axis to impair visual acuity.

The cornea may exhibit a keratitis or dystrophy, edema or vascularization or a more advanced keratoconus.

The lens may be cataractous, luxated or subluxated.

Any component of the uveal tract (iris, ciliary body, choroid) can cause visual impairment in an inflammatory or hemorrhagic condition and also with tumors.

The vitreous if involved in an inflammatory or hemorrhagic condition will easily impair visual acuity.

Many pathological conditions involving the retina must be considered in the evaluation of poor visual acuity. These conditions include vascular occlusion, serous retinopathy, any of the macular degeneration or tapetoretinal degeneration, retinitis (chorioretinitis), toxic amblyopia, tumors, exposure to infrared radiation (eclipse of the sun), and retinal detachment.

The optic nerve if involved in an inflammatory tumor or atrophic condition certainly will cause visual impairment. Interestingly, papilledema does not cause changes in visual acuity until an advanced stage.

PHOTOPHOBIA OR GLARE WITH OR WITHOUT TEARING

This is ocular discomfort with exposure to bright light. Causes include a dilated, nonreactive pupil; light uveal pigmentation, i. e., albinism, blunt corneal trauma or keratitis; corneal edema; iritis; and in infants congenital glaucoma.

POOR VISION IN DIM LIGHT

This is often expressed as difficulty seeing at night. This is often the first complaint in a person with retinitis pigmentosa (pigmentary retinal degeneration) but may often be found in people with a vitamin A deficiency and in some with myopia.

DISTORTED VISION

This is a condition in which objects are either irregular, micropsic, or macropsic as a result of a condition which causes macular edema such as commotio retinae (from blunt trauma), central serous retinopathy, or flat retinal detachment.

LOSS OF PERIPHERAL VISION

In this condition a person complains of bumping into things or having a shade or curtain covering his side vision. Possible causes are partial retinal detachment, vitreoretinal hemorrhages or, more commonly, central nervous system disease (vascular or neoplastic).

SPOTS IN FRONT OF THE EYE

A common complaint of myopes and older persons caused by the breakdown of the normal vitreous gel into liquified pockets containing strands of vitreous which cast shadows, a condition referred to as "floaters." A tear in the retina may release a small amount of hemorrhage which presents as a spot or spots. Synchisis scintillans or deposits of cholesterol in the vitreous may cast shadows and cause spots to be seen.

SPOTS OR FLASHES OF LIGHT

These can be caused by involvement of the retina, optic nerve or central nervous system, blunt trauma to the globe, or occipital lobe migraine, impending retinal detachment or Moore's lightning flashes, often present with a complaint of having seen lights flashing.

DOUBLE VISION OR DIPLOPIA

In this condition an individual sees two of everything. Most frequently it is caused by misalignment of the visual axes, because of muscle or innervation abnormalities, such as ocular muscle paresis in diabetes, peripheral nerve degeneration, or entrapment in orbital fractures. Children with ocular deviations do not complain of diplopia because of their ability to mentally suppress one of the images, a condition that creates another problem, known as amblyopia ex anopsia. Monocular diplopia in reality requires two openings in the iris to cause two distinct separate images or true diplopia. Some of the monocular conditions often interpreted as blurred vision and not diplopia can be caused by an astigmatic cornea or lenticular changes.

RINGS OR COLORED HALOES AROUND LIGHTS

This is most often caused by a condition which leads to corneal edema, most importantly, acute-angle closure glaucoma. Other corneal problems such as opacities, scars, dystrophies, or movement of conjunctional secretions across the cornea plus opacification of the lens may cause this sensation.

CHANGES IN COLOR VISION

A condition creating either an intensification of a color or a change to a different color occurs here. This is a probable complaint caused by a "normal" physiologic response depending on background lighting, nuclear sclerosis, or postoperative cataract extraction.

MOVING OBJECTS OR OBJECT SEEM TO MOVE IN FRONT OF ME

These are all complaints of a form of vertigo. Ocular causes can result from a vertical muscle imbalance or a peripheral nerve innervation defect to the extraocular muscles or the first wearing of new glasses, especially the first pair of bifocals. Nonocular causes should include labyrinth disturbance and central nervous system disease.

COMPLAINTS WITHOUT A VISUAL COMPONENT

FOREIGN BODY SENSATION

This is a common, nonvisual ocular complaint caused by anything that disrupts the corneal epithelium such as corneal abrasion, corneal foreign body, foreign body lodged under the upper lid, superficial keratitis or vernal conjunctivitis, entropian, cilia lodged in a punctum, trichiasis, corneal blebs, edema, and dystrophies which demonstrate breakdown in the epithelial layer of the cornea.

ACHING, THROBBING OCULAR, PERIOCULAR PAIN AND/OR HEADACHES

These usually are symptoms indicative of an injury or inflammation of the anterior uvea such as iritis, iridocyclitis, herpes zoster, and tic douloureux. However, other conditions, such as sinusitis, orbital abscess, retrobulbar neuritis or central nervous system (CNS) vascularization, or aneurysm, can create this discomfort with refined pain.

HEADACHES

Interestingly, headaches are rarely caused because of an ocular problem. More often there is a nonocular cause such as sinusitis, hypertension, migraine, or central nervous system (CNS) vasculitis. Ocular conditions which may present as a headache are uncorrected refractive error, EOM muscle imbalance, chronic open-angle glaucoma, acute-angle closure glaucoma, and inflammation of the anterior uvea.

TENDERNESS

This is usually an indication of inflammation of periorbital tissues such as the lid, i. e. , blepharitis, hordeolum, cellulitis, the lacrimal gland (dacryoadenitis), the lacrimal sac (dacryocystitis), orbital cellulitis, or abscess and refined pain from any source, i. e. , sinusitis. Ocular causes producing tenderness are conditions such as corneal abrasions and foreign bodies, episcleritis, iritis, or iridocyclitis.

BURNING

This is a vague symptom often referred to as smarting and is found in conditions such as the dry eye syndrome, e. g. ,

Sjogren's syndrome, uncorrected refractive error, conjunctivitis or keratitis, exposure to wind, dust, pollen, and other irritants, and insufficient sleep.

DULL ACHING OR DRAWING SENSATION

This is a fairly common complaint, especially in people who are required to do a lot of reading, e. g., medical school students, and is due to either an uncorrected refractive error or extraocular muscle imbalance, especially vertical, or convergence insufficiency.

EXCESSIVE TEARING OR EPIPHORIA

This may be caused by excessive tear formation secondary to abnormal tear production, inflammation, i. e., conjunctivitis, blockage in the lacrimal drainage system (canaliculus, lacrimal sac, or nasolacrimal duct), exposure to excessive light, to wind or to atmospheric irritants, e. g., smoke, or to a disturbed emotional state.

ITCHY EYE

This condition is frequently found in allergic conjunctivitis and when the patient is tired or strained. It is also a condition created as wounds heal.

DRY EYE SYNDROME

This is most frequently found in older persons and arthritics caused by either an insufficient tear formation or the formation of altered abnormal tears. A dryness sensation is also present in people with malpositioned lids or those that have improper lid closure, i. e., Graves' disease. Often associated with the dryness is the sensation of grittiness or a sandy feeling caused by the presence of dried secretion.

EYE TWITCHING

This condition is often an indication of generalized fatigue. It is called a tic and is unilateral.

LIDS FEEL HEAVY

This is another sign of generalized fatigue but may also be found when there is a lid inflammation, e. g., hordeolum, or edema, e. g. , allergic reaction of the upper lids. Ptosis in myasthenia gravis and blepharochalasia also present with heavy lid symptoms.

BULGING EYE

If this complaint is of recent onset, it may be an indication of more serious problems. The exophthalmos may be caused by an orbital mass, i. e. , abscess, tumor, hemorrhage. It may be an indication of thyroid disease or the result of lid retraction found in thyroid disease, hypertension, or meningiomas.

FREQUENT OR EXCESSIVE BLINKING

This may be associated with a facial tic or result from local irritation, e. g. , foreign body, misdirected cilia.

SQUINTING OR NARROWING OF THE PALPEBRAL FISSURE

This is a mechanism used to either reduce the amount of light entering the eye, e. g. , reduce glare, or correct a refractive error, especially in myopes, by creating the pinhole effect of the old box cameras.

LIDS STUCK TOGETHER

This is usually associated with an inflammatory or infectious condition, e. g. , conjunctivitis, and is caused by the drying of secreted material (e. g. , mucous or pus) on the lid margins and lashes.

WHITE MATTER IN THE CORNER OF THE EYE

This may be related to an infectious process, but more often is associated with an overactive meibomian gland which releases an oily substance as a part of the tear formation.

GRANULATED EYELIDS

This is a collection of dried secretions in the cilia and margin indicative of an inflammatory process, e. g. , blepharitis, most often caused by staphylococci or seborrhea.

DIZZINESS

This is seldom caused by an eye disorder other than an uncorrected refractive error, heterophoria, and most likely the unaccustomed us of new eye glasses, especially the first pair of bifocals. More often the examination should be directed toward the vestibular and cerebellar systems.

APPENDIX II: COMMONLY USED DRUGS IN OPHTHALMOLOGY

A. ANTIGLAUCOMA DROPS

Drug	Concentration	Doses	Color of Top
Epinephrine	1, 2%	b.i.d.	White
Bitartrate	1, 2%		
Hydrochloride	0.25, 0.5, 1, 2%		
Borate	0.25, 0.5, 1%		
Dipivefrin Hydrochloride (Propine)	0.1%		
Timolol Maleate (Timoptic)	0.25%	b.i.d.	Blue
	0.5%	b.i.d.	Yellow

Adverse Reactions	Systemic Effects	Note
Caution in narrow-angle glaucoma. Local allergic reactions. Adrenochrome deposits. Reversible macula edema in aphakic patients. Soft contact lens wearers, lens may turn black.	Alpha and beta stimulator. Caution in patients with hypertensive, cardiovascular, or coronary artery disease.	Increases facility of outflow. Propine is a pro-drug that becomes active after entering the eye. This should account for less local and systemic side effects.
Allergic reactions. Very few local side effects.	Beta 1 and beta 2 adrenergic blocker. Contraindicated in bronchial asthma, 2nd or 3rd degree heart block, bradycardia, diabetes—symptoms of hypoglycemia may be marked.	At present major action believed to be reduction of aqueous production.

A. Antiglaucoma Drops (Cont'd)

Drug	Concentration	Doses	Color of Top
Miotics			
Pilocarpine Hydrochloride	0.25-10%	q.i.d.	Green
Pilocarpine Epinephrine Combination	P1% P2 P3 P4 P6	q.i.d.	Green
Carbachol	0.75, 1.5, 2.25, 3%	t.i.d. or q.i.d.	Green
Echothiophate Iodide (Phospholine Iodide)	0.03, 0.06, 0.125, 0.25%	q.i.d. or b.i.d.	Green

Adverse Reactions	Systemic Effects	Note
Miosis-reduced visual acuity in poor illumination. Supraorbital headache-induced myopia.	Cholinergic parasympathomimetic. Systemic side effects are rare but may occur in overdose. See pharmacology text for cholinergic systemic effects.	Miosis of iris which puts tension on the scleral spur, thus opening the trabecular meshwork.
Same as pilocarpine and epinephrine	Same as pilocarpine and epinephrine	
Same as pilocarpine	See pharmacology text for cholinesterase inhibitors.	Partially inhibits cholinesterase.
Both plasma and erythrocyte levels of cholinesterase will be lowered after a few weeks of use. Patients on echothiophate iodide should be cautioned about general anesthesia, because of inability to reverse effects of succinylcholine. Caution in patients under treatment for myasthenia gravis with systemic cholinesterase inhibitors.		Not used as primary drug for glaucoma. Pilocarpine is better and has less toxic effects. Used in children for diagnosis of accommodative esotropia.

A. Antiglaucoma Drops (Cont'd)

Drug	Concentration	Doses	Color of Top
Demecarium Bromide (Humorsol)	0.125, 0.25%	Twice a week to b.i.d.	Green
Diisopropyl phosphoro-fluroidate (DFP)	0.025% ointment		
Physostigmine (Eserine)	0.25% ointment 0.25, 0.5% solution		

Adverse Reactions	Systemic Effects	Note
Iris cysts, especially in children. Will disappear with discontinuance of medication.		Very infrequently used. Not a primary drug.
Longest acting cholinesterase inhibitor		Not used for glaucoma having been replaced by phospholine iodide. Mostly used in children with accommodative esotropia.
		Seldom used for glaucoma, has been helpful in treating pediculosis and phthiriasis of the eye lashes.

B. TOPICAL ANTIBACTERIALS

Drug	Preparation
Bacitracin	500 μ/g ointment
Chloramphenicol	0.5% drops
(Chloromycetin) (Chloroptic) (Econochlor) (Ophthochlor)	1.0% ointment
Erythromycin (Ilotycin)	0.5% ointment
Gentamycin Sulfate (Garamycin) (Genoptic)	3 mg/ml drops and ointment
Sulfacetamide Sodium	15% drops 10% ointment
(Bleph-10) (Cetamide) (Isoptocetamide) (Sulamyd) (Sulfasel-15) (Vasosulf)	
Sulfisoxozale Dialamine (Gantrisin)	4% drops Ointment

Major Spectrum for Ophthalmic Use	Note
Gram-positive cocci and bacilli	Very limited ophthalmic use.
Gram-positive cocci and bacilli Some gram-negative	Bacteriostatic, should not be used in combination with bacteriocidal antibiotics. Aplastic anemia has been reported with use of ophthalmic preparations.
Chlamydial inclusion conjunctivitis. Trachoma	Chlamydial infections should be treated both orally and topically.
Gram-negative rods	Aminoglycosides are drugs of choice for serious ocular infections and corneal ulcers. Fortified gentamycin can be made by mixing 80 mg/ml injectable gentamycin with bottle of drops.
Gram-positive cocci	Most preferred initial therapy for mild to moderate conjunctivitis.

B. Topical Antibacterial (Cont'd)

Drug	Preparation
Tetracycline (Achromycin) (Aureomycin)	1% drops and ointment
Tobramycin (Tobex)	0.3% drops and ointment
Mixture	
Chloramphenicol and Polymyxin B (Chloromyxin)	1% + 10,000 μ/g
Polymyxin + Neomycin Sulfate Bacitracin (Mycitracin) (Neosporin)	5000 μ + 5 mg + 500 μ/g
Polymyxin B + Bacitracin (Polysporin)	10,000 μ + 5 μ/g
Neomycin + Polymyxin B (Stratal)	3.5 mg + 10,000 μ/g
Polymyxin B + Oxytetracycline (Terramycin/ Polymyxin)	10,000 μ + 30 mg/g

Major Spectrum for Ophthalmic Use	Note
Chlamydial trachoma	Drug of choice. Treatment both systemic and topical.
Same as gentamycin	See gentamycin
	Combination ophthalmic preparations have gained popularity among ophthalmologists. They give no better coverage than non-mixture preparations. Neomycin is also highly allergenic.

C. MYDRIATICS—RED TOP

Drug	Concen-tration	Duration of Action	Desired Ophthalmic Effect
Mydriatic Only			
Phenylephrine Hydrochloride (Neosynephrine)	2.5, 10% drops	2-3 hr	Pupillary dilation. Treatment of uveitis. Refraction. Fundus examination. Vasoconstriction. Ocular decongestant.
Cycloplegic, mydriatic			
Tropicamide (Mydriacyl)	0.5, 1% drops	2-6 hr	Pupillary dilation and cycloplegia, uveitis, refraction, fundus examination
Cyclopentolate Hydrochloride (Cyclogyl)	0.5, 1, 2% drops	3-8 hr	Same as tropicamide
Homatropine Hydrobromide	2, 5% drops	2-4 hr	Long duration pupillary dilation, cycloplegia, uveitis, refraction, in children
Scopolamine Hydrobromide (Hyocine)	0.25% drops	4-7 days	Same as homatropine

Contra-indications	Side Effects and Adverse Reactions	Note
Narrow-angle glaucoma. 10% in unstable. Hypertension or cardiac patients. Known sensitivity to phenylephrine	Glare in sunlight. Transient blurred vision.	Direct action on pupillary dilator muscle. No cycloplegic effect. 2.5% is safer.
Narrow-angle glaucoma	Loss of accommodation in young individuals. Psychotic changes, photophobia, dry mouth.	Anticholinergic, blocks sphincter muscle.
Narrow-angle glaucoma	Same as tropicamide, psychotic and behavioral changes common in elderly and young children.	Same as tropicamide.
Narrow-angle glaucoma	2-4 days loss accommodation (reading vision), photophobia, dry mouth.	Anticholinergic moderate to long duration.
Narrow-angle glaucoma	Same as homatropine but 4-7 days duration.	Same as homatropine.

C. Mydriatics—Red Top (Cont'd)

Drug	Concen-tration	Duration of Action	Desired Ophthalmic Effect
Atropine Sulfate	0.5, 1, 3% drops 1% ointment	7-14 days	Same as homatropine

Contra-indications	Side Effects and Adverse Reactions	Note
Narrow-angle glaucoma	Same as homatropine but up to 2 weeks duration	Patients will commonly present to emergency room after using someone else's drops. Complaint will be blurred vision, photophobia, inability to read. If dilated pupils do not react to light, or 0.5% pilocarpine, suspect atropine or other cycloplegics. Hospital personnel in emergency room with dilated pupils and loss of accommodation, r/o atropine.

D. CARBONIC ANHYDRASE INHIBITORS

Drug	Mg	Dose
Acetazolamide (Diamox)	125, 250 mg tabs	Up to q. i. d.
	500 mg sequals	Up to b. i. d.
Injection	250-500 mg 5-10 ml	IM or IV 500 mg/12 hr
Methazolamide (Neptazane)	50 mg tabs	b. i. d. or t. i. d.
Dichlorphenamide (Daranide)	50 mg tabs	q. d. b. i, d. or t. i. d.

Adverse Reactions	Note
Nonbacteriostatic sulfonamide contraindicated in patients allergic to sulfonamides	In emergency room setting for therapy of acute-angle closure glaucoma.
See pharmacology text for all side effects of sulfonamides	Few adverse reactions will be seen.
May precipitate or aggravate acidosis paresthesia (tingling of extremities)	
Long-term therapy chance of nephrolithiasis	
Diuretic effect, caution with electrolytes	
Similar to Diamox	In emergency room Diamox better for acute-angle closure.
Same side effects, may be of less intensity	Neptazane may be better in simple open-angle glaucoma for chronic carbonic anhydrase inhibitor therapy.
Similar to all carbonic anhydrase inhibitors	All carbonic anhydrase inhibitors seem to work by decreasing aqueous production at the level of the ciliary body.

E. HYPEROSMOTIC AGENTS

Drug	Route of Administration	Dosage
Glycerin (Glyrol)	Oral	75% solution 1.0-1.5 g/kg q. 6-8 hr 1 ml-0.94 g
(Osmoglyn)		50% solution
Mannitol (Osmitrol)	IV	20% solution 1.5-2 g/kg 30-60 min
Isosobide Solution (Isonal) (Hydronal)	Oral	45% solution 1.5 g/kg
Urea	IV	30% solution 1-1.5 g/kg

Adverse Reactions	Note
Caution in diabetics, elderly, dehydrated individuals Nausea, vomiting, dehydration, confusion, disorientation	Oral osmotic agent indicated in acute-angle closure glaucoma when nausea is not present. If not flavored give over ice with orange or lemon juice.
Causes acute expansion of extracellular fluid. Not to be used in patients with pulmonary edema or congestive heart failure.	Used in acute-angle closure glaucoma not responding to therapy with miotics, carbonic anhydrase inhibitors or glycerine.
Similar to glycerine. Diuresis is greater.	May be of value in brittle diabetics because it does not cause hyperglycemia
Urea is very irritating if extravasation occurs. Thrombosis and pain can occur.	Very little use today because of the problem with extravasation.

F. OCULAR DECONGESTANTS

Drug	Trade Names
Naphazoline Hydrochloride	Albalon Clear Eyes Degest 2 Naphcon Opcon Vasoclear Vasocon Regulor
Phenylephrine Hydrochloride	Efricel Isoptofrin Prefrin
Tetrahydrozoline Hydrochloride	Murine Sooth Visine

G. OCULAR LUBRICANTS (Artificial Tears)

Adapettes	Liquifilm Forte
Adsorbotear	Liquifilm Tears
aqua-FLOW	Liquifilm Wetting Solution
Clertz	Lyteers
Comfort Drops	Methopto
Dual Wet	Methulose
hy-FLOW	Murocel
Hypotears	Neo-Tears
Isopto Alkaline	Pre-Sert
Isopto Plain	Tearisol
Isopto Tears	Tears Naturale
Lacril	Tears Plus*
Lacrisert*	Total
(Water soluble insert)	Visculose
Lens-Mate	Wetting Solution
Lensine 5	

*Prescription medication; all the other preparations are non-prescription.

Ophthalmic Uses	Note
All drugs of this type are whitening agents. Sometimes used in combination with antibiotics in conjunctivitis for psychological effect.	All drugs of this type may have rebound hyperemia, especially when used frequently.
	When the trade names have an A following them, they are decongestants with antihistamine. Used mainly for ocular allergy (hay fever, vernal catarrh).
Dry Eye Syndrome Sjögren's Syndrome Keratoconjunctivitis Sicca Stevens-Johnson Syndrome Chemical Burns	

H. TOPICAL OCULAR ANESTHETIC AGENTS

Drug	Concentration
Proparacaine Hydrochloride (Alcaine) (Opththaine) (Ophthetic)	0.5% solution
Tetracaine Hydrochloride (Ancel) (Pontocaine)	0.5% solution
Cocaine	Solutions made by pharmacy 1%, 4%, 10%

Adverse Reactions	Note
Transient local symptoms, rarely acute allergic reaction with keratitis and sloughing of corneal epithelium.	All topical ophthalmic anesthetics are used short term—examination and procedures. A patient should never be prescribed or given any of these medications. Prolonged use may lead to diminished healing or worse infections.

I. ANTIVIRAL ANTIHERPETIC

Drug	Preparation	Dose
Idoxuridine (I. D. U.) (Dendrid) (Herplex)	0. 1% Drops	q. 1 hr to q. 4 hr
(Stoxil)	0. 1% Drops or 0. 5% ointment	
Vidarabine (Vira-A)	3% Ointment	5 times a day
Trifluridine (Viroptic)	1% Solution	5 times a day to q. 2 hr

Adverse Reactions	Note
Irritation, pruritis, edema or photophobia. Superficial punctate staining of cornea.	Action: irreversibly inhibits incorporation of thymidire into viral DNA
Lacrimation, foreign body sensation, superficial punctate staining of cornea.	Appears to interfere with early DNA synthesis
Same as the other antivirals.	Interferes with DNA synthesis. Mechanism not completely known. None of the antivirals are recommended for pregnant women. Vidarabine and trifluridine have shown teratogenic potential in animals.

J. OCULAR CORTICOSTEROIDS

Drug	Concentration
Hydrocortisone	
(Hydrocortisone Acetate)	2.5% suspension
	1.5% ointment
(Optef)	0.2% solution
Prednisolone	0.125-1.0% suspension
(Econopred/Econopred Plus)	
(Hydeltrasol)	0.5% solution
	0.25% ointment
(Inflamase Forte)	0.12-1.0% solution
(Metreton)	0.5% solution
(Pred Mild/Forte)	0.12-1.0% suspension
(Predulose)	0.25% suspension
Dexamethasone	0.1% solution
(Decadron)	0.5% ointment
(Maxidex)	0.1% suspension
Pogesterone-like	1.0% solution
Medrysone	0.1% suspension

Ophthalmic Uses	Note
Uveitis Ocular inflammatory Ocular allergy Vernal conjunctivitis	Ocular steroids should not be prescribed routinely. Patients using corticosteroids must be followed by an ophthalmologist. Susceptible individuals may develop glaucoma. Prolonged use can cause cataracts. Herpes simplex may be exacerbated or new attacks started.

K. CORTICOSTEROID—ANTIBACTERIAL PREPARATIONS

Drug	Trade Names
Corticosteroid/ Sulfonamide Suspensions and Ointments	Blephamide Cetapred Isopto Cetapred Ocu-lone-C Predsulfair Sulphrin
Corticosteroid/ Chloramphenicol	Chloromycetin/Hydrocortisone Chloroptic P-SOP
Corticosteroid/Polymyxin B/ Neomycin	Cortisporin Dexasporin Maxitrol Poly-Pred Ocu-Spor-B Ocutrol
Corticosteroid/Neomycin	NeoDecadron
Corticosteroid/Neomycin/ Bacitracin/Polymyxin	Ocutricin

Ophthalmic Uses	Note
Blepharitis Conjunctivitis Keratitis Postoperative	Should not be used routinely for conjunctivitis because of problems discussed under corticosteroids.

APPENDIX III: DISC SWELLING—DIFFERENTIAL DIAGNOSIS

1. Papilledema—Elevated Intracranial Pressure
   (See Appendices IV and V)

2. Ocular Disease
   - A. Hypotomy
   - B. Uveitis
   - C. Trauma

3. Vascular Disease
   - A. Nonarteritic Ischemic Neuropathy (ION)
   - B. Arteritic ION
     1. Cranial Artents
     2. Collagen Vascular Disease
   - C. Diabetic Papillopathy

4. Inflammatory Disease
   - A. Papillitis

5. Orbital Disease
   - A. Tumor
     1. Meningioma
     2. Glioma
     3. Metastatic
   - B. Thyroid Ophthalmopathy

6. Meningeal
   - A. Meningitis
   - B. Infiltrative swelling
     1. Leukemia
     2. Lymphoma
     3. Carcinomatosis

7. Systemic Disease
   A. Hypertension
   B. Anemia
   C. Hypovolemia
   D. Hypoxemia (pulmonary)
   E. Sarcoidosis

APPENDIX IV: PAPILLEDEMA—CAUSES OF INCREASED INTRACRANIAL PRESSURE

1. Intracranial Mass
    A. Tumor (especially posterior fossa)
    B. Brain abscess
    C. Subdural hematoma

2. Pseudotumor Cerebri

3. Meningeal
    A. Meningitis
    B. Subarachnoid hemorrhage
    C. Meningeal Carcinomatosis

4. Vascular
    A. Hypertension
    B. Cerebral Venous Sinus Thrombus
    C. Radical Neck Dissection
    D. Congestive Heart Failure
    E. Superior Vena Cava Syndrome

5. Developmental
    A. Hydrocephalus
    B. Craniostenosis

6. Toxic
    A. Vitamin A
    B. Tetracycline
    C. Nalidixic Acid

Toxic (continued)

- D. Steroids
- E. Lead Poisoning

7. Systemic Disease
   - A. Uremia
   - B. Lupus Erythematosus
   - C. Sarcoidosis
   - D. Leukemia
   - E. Polycythemia
   - F. Diabetic Ketacidosis

APPENDIX V: SYMPTOMS AND SIGNS OF INCREASED INTRACRANIAL PRESSURE

A. Symptoms
   1. Systemic
      a. Headache
      b. Nausea and Vomiting
      c. Dizziness

   2. Ocular
      a. Transient Visual Obscurations (less than 30 seconds)
      b. Binocular Diplopia

B. Signs
   1. Systemic
      a. Bradycardia and Hypotension
      b. Respiratory Changes

   2. Ocular
      a. Papilledema
      b. Abducens Nerve Palsy
      c. Oculomotor Nerve Palsy (suggests herniation)
      d. Visual field constriction with blind spot enlargement.

APPENDIX VI: CAUSES OF PSEUDOPAPILLEDEMA

1. Drusen (hyaline bodies) of optic nerve
2. Hyperopia
3. Myelinated Nerve Fibers
4. Hyaloid Remnants ("gliosis")
5. Dysplasia of Optic Disc
6. Disc Neoplasms

INDEX